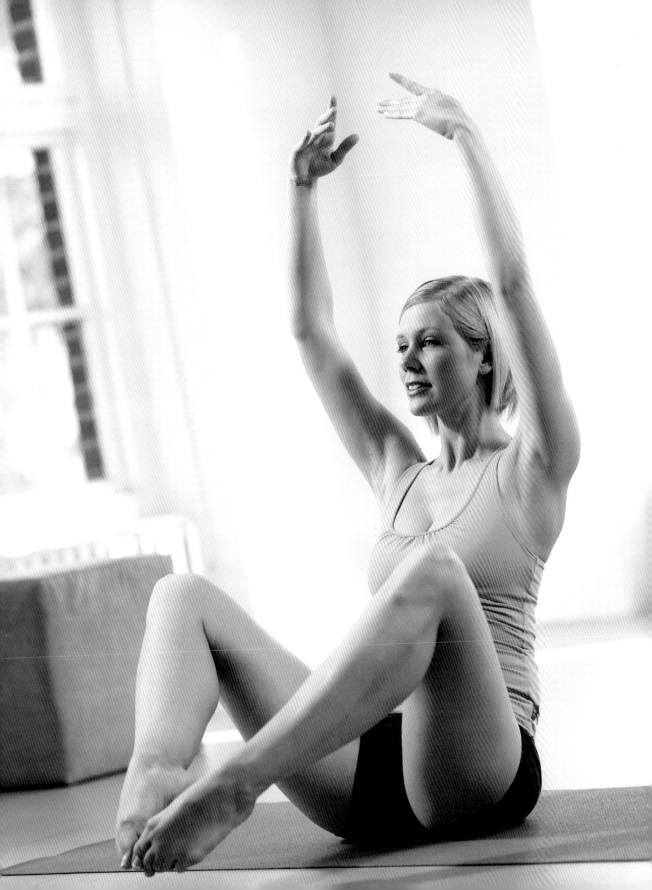

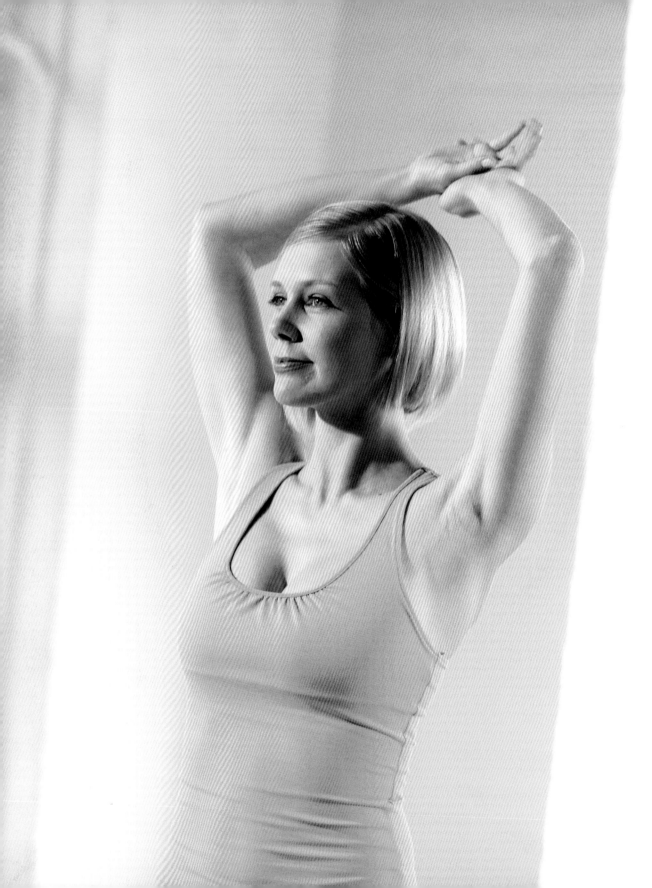

>> **15**minute

better back
workout

Suzanne Martin P.T., D.P.T.

London, New York, Melbourne, Munich, and Delhi

For Michael Smuin, choreographer extraordinaire
and a peach of a guy

Project Editor Hilary Mandleberg
Project Art Director Miranda Harvey
Senior Art Editor Peggy Sadler
Managing Editor Penny Warren
Managing Art Editor Marianne Markham
Art Director Peter Luff
Publishing Director Mary-Clare Jerram
Stills Photography Ruth Jenkinson
DTP Designer Sonia Charbonnier
Production Controllers Rebecca Short, Sarah Sherlock
Production Editor Luca Frassinetti
Jacket Designer Neal Cobourne

DVD produced for Dorling Kindersley by
Chrome Productions www.chromeproductions.com

Director Robin Schmidt
DOP Marcus Domleo, Matthew Cooke
Camera Joe McNally, Marcus Domleo, Jonathan Iles
Production Manager Hannah Chandler
Production Assistant Azra Gul
Grip Pete Nash
Gaffer Paul Wilcox, Johann Cruickshank
Music Chad Hobson
Hair and Makeup Victoria Barnes
Voiceover Suzanne Pirret
Voiceover Recording Ben Jones

First American Edition, 2008

Published in the United States by
DK Publishing
375 Hudson Street
New York, New York 10014

08 09 10 11 10 9 8 7 6 5 4 3 2

ND091/Jan-08

Published in Great Britain by Dorling Kindersley Limited.

A catalog record for this book is available from
the Library of Congress

ISBN 978-07566-2856-7

DK books are available at special discounts when
purchased in bulk for sales promotions, premiums, fund-
raising, or educational use. For details, contact:
DK Publishing Special Markets, 375 Hudson Street,
New York, New York 10014 or SpecialSales@dk.com.

Health warning
Always consult your doctor before starting a fitness program
if you have any health concerns, and especially if you are
pregnant, have given birth in the last six weeks, or have a
medical condition such as high blood pressure, arthritis, or
asthma. This book is not intended for people suffering from
back problems; it provides programs to strengthen the back
and prevent back problems from occurring. If you have any
pain while exercising, stop immediately.

Every effort has been made to ensure that the information
contained in this book is complete and accurate. However,
neither the publisher nor the author is engaged in rendering
professional advice or services to the individual reader. The
ideas, information, and suggestions contained in this book
are not intended as a substitute for consulting with your
physician. All matters regarding your health require medical
supervision. Neither the author nor the publisher shall be
liable or responsible for any loss or damage allegedly rising
from any information or suggestion in this book.

Printed and bound by Sheck Wah Tong, China

Discover more at
www.dk.com

contents

author foreword

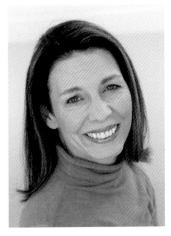

Congratulations on buying this book and embarking on the road to your better back! I'm pleased to share with you the exercises, knowledge, and techniques that have helped me, as well as countless others, in my classes, courses, and private practice for over 25 years.

All of us need a better back. My own back has a special story. I've had minor scoliosis throughout my whole active career as a dancer, dance and exercise instructor, Pilates expert, and physical therapist. It's likely that you need help, too, since studies show that nearly 80 percent of all people will suffer from some type of back problem in their lifetimes. This book contains tips and exercises to help you avoid and, if necessary, alleviate most common back episodes.

Life is imperfect; nature is imperfect. Look at the leaves on a tree. See how they are each shaped slightly differently and how each has countless imperfections in texture and shape. Our bodies reflect nature's imperfections, which means that we all have our own set of physical nuances, and that includes the back. Daily wear and tear makes it essential for all of us to acquire a better back. Lifting children and groceries, gardening, running, climbing—even sitting too long—can all lead to a sore back. Learning proper posture and the preventive exercises in this book can contribute, on a daily basis, to giving us an improved quality of life, which, now that we are all living longer, is more important than ever.

Exercising and learning new techniques and concepts increases body awareness so you get greater control over your physicality, but there are other benefits, too. Your resiliency against life's knocks and falls will improve. Strengthening your neck gives confidence to your voice. Nurturing your upper and mid-back allows your heart to risk the perils of love. Reinforcing your lower back will help you stay firm in your resolve. These are the mind–body connections that you often hear people speak of. If you feel confident and resilient in your body, your mind will reflect those qualities as well. *Better Back Workout* is a powerful gateway to all of this. Enjoy.

Suzanne Martin

>> **how to use** this book

This book promises a better back! First take time to study the exercises in detail and familiarize yourself with what you will need to do. Each exercise is valid by itself but, when you follow the correct sequence, the magic happens. Let me help you see the forest as well as the trees.

Each of my programs focuses on a different way of working the back. The accompanying DVD is designed to be used with the book to reinforce the exercises shown there. As you watch the DVD, page references to the book flash up on the screen. Refer to these for more detailed instruction. In the book, the exercises each have a beginning position, shown in the inset, and two successive parts. Annotations give you tips on proper positioning, and white dotted-line "feel-it-here" patches home in on specific body areas. Not all pictures have these since a number of exercises are concerned with the whole body.

Some exercises are more difficult than others. The programs build to a crescendo of intensity, then gently back away. The first exercises in each program are warm-ups and mobility exercises. The next are often stretches, and are followed by abdominal exercises. Then come the harder back and full-body exercises, and finally the sequence ends on a softer note. Even beginners should be able to do most of the exercises. For tips on how often to perform the programs, how to modify the exercises if needed, and how to combine them for a longer workout, see pp. 116–117.

The gatefolds

The gatefolds help you see each *Better Back Workout* program in full view. Once you've watched the DVD and examined each exercise, use the gatefolds as a quick reference to trim your exercise time down to a succinct 15 minutes.

Safety issues

Be sure to get clearance from your healthcare provider prior to beginning any exercise program. The advice and exercises here are not intended to be a substitute for individual medical help. Your medical specialist may recommend preparatory exercises especially tailored to your needs.

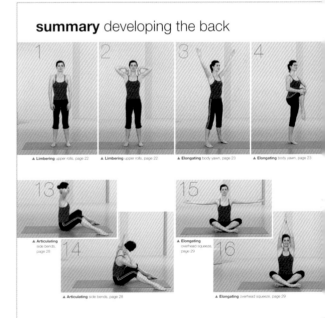

summary developing the back

1 ▲ Limbering upper rolls, page 22
2 ▲ Limbering upper rolls, page 22
3 ▲ Elongating body yawn, page 23
4 ▲ Elongating body yawn, page 23
13 ▲ Articulating side bends, page 28
14 ▲ Articulating side bends, page 28
15 ▲ Elongating overhead squeeze, page 29
16 ▲ Elongating overhead squeeze, page 29

Gatefold The gatefold gives you a comprehensive demonstration of the entire program—an easy reference to make your workout quick and simple.

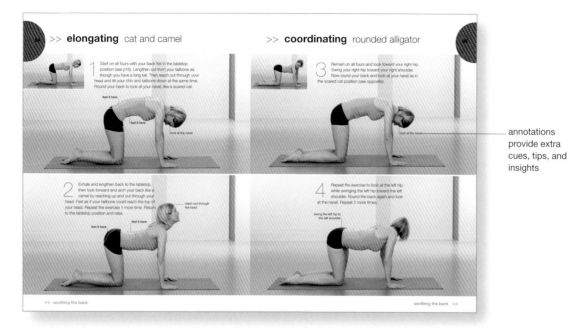

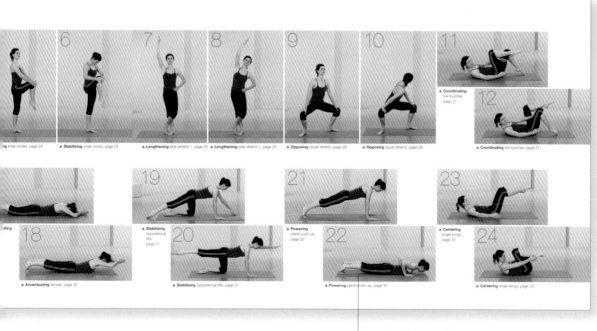

annotations provide extra cues, tips, and insights

Step-by-step pages The inset photograph at the upper left gives you the starting position for the exercise. The next two photographs show the steps required to complete it.

the gatefold shows all the main steps of the program

>> **the parts of** the back

Take a moment at this point to review the four different parts of the back.

Each has a different role to play in enabling us to perform our everyday tasks.

Getting a clear idea of the four main sections of your back will help you to

make your exercises more effective. Look in the mirror and follow along.

The "back" is technically the "spine" and is made up of several parts. Looking from the side, it makes a long S-curve. The spine has four main curves: the cervical, the thoracic, the lumbar, and the fused sacral/coccyx. The curves are not present at birth and only begin to develop when an infant achieves vertical standing and at toddler stage when he or she begins to walk. The downward press of gravity shapes the spine and gives each curve an all-important role in maintaining the health of the back and producing bipedal stance.

The cervical spine

The cervical spine or upper neck can be felt at your hairline, just at the base of the skull. It is responsible for tipping the chin upward and downward. The upper part of the cervical spine also contains the muscles responsible for eye motions. If you keep your fingertips at the base and dart your eyes back and forth, you'll detect the motions of these fine muscles.

The lower cervical spine is convex-shaped. You can usually feel the prominent southernmost vertebra as it meets the shoulders. The neck has the greatest amount of range of motion of the spine. It can create a telescoping effect and can swivel to almost look completely behind you.

The thoracic spine

This has a concave shape and is connected with the rib cage. You can trace the prominent spinous processes, the visible bumps of the spine, by

> ## >> **the four main** parts of the back
>
> - **The cervical spine,** or "neck," has seven vertebrae and extends from the base of the skull to the shoulders.
>
> - **The thoracic spine,** comprising the upper and mid-back, has 12 vertebrae and extends from the shoulders to the waist.
>
> - **The lumbar spine,** or "lower back," has five vertebrae. This vulnerable section forms the waist and has no bony support.
>
> - **The sacral section** contains the four fused vertebrae of the sacrum with the vestigial tail, the "coccyx," at its end.

running your thumbs from your shoulders down to the top of your waist. It is chronically stiff since it's girdled by the rib cage, so developing mobility in the thoracic spine requires patience.

The lumbar spine

Put your hands around your waist to find the lumbar spine. This part of the spine is particularly vulnerable because it's balancing the weight of the trunk against the unwieldy weighty legs. What's special about the lumbar spine is its springboard effect on the spine. Its convex shape allows the impact against the ground to dissipate as you step.

The back is not a single entity but is actually made up of four main sections. The exercises in *Better Back Workout* will help you strengthen each of them.

The curves make an S-shape that gives the back resilience. Preserving those curves is all-important if you want a pain-free back!

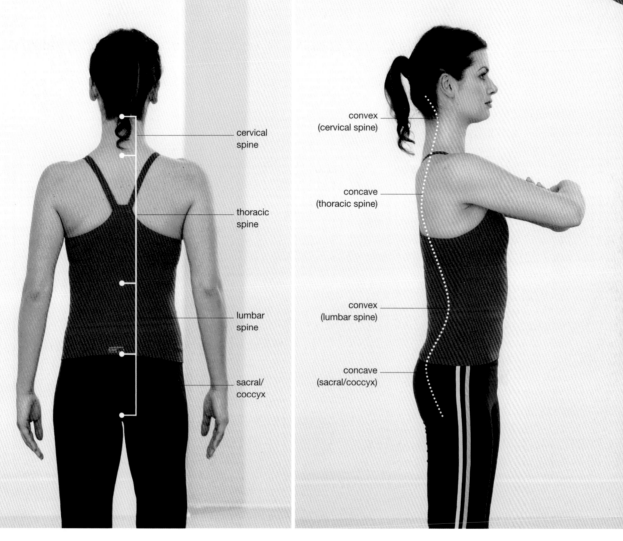

cervical spine

thoracic spine

lumbar spine

sacral/ coccyx

convex (cervical spine)

concave (thoracic spine)

convex (lumbar spine)

concave (sacral/coccyx)

The sacrum

Finally, place your hands on your hip bones, fingers facing forward, and your thumbs will end up on top of the fused vertebrae of the sacrum. Very large forces converge here—at the sacroiliac joints—the place where the lumbar spine and the sacrum meet. That means that this area is extremely vulnerable and requires careful positioning and handling if you are to avoid injury. At the bottom of this fusion lies the coccyx or tailbone.

The discs

These are pieces of cartilage that lie between the vertebrae. Think of them as being like jelly donuts, with a soft center and a hard exterior. They provide cushioning in between the vertebrae but, even more importantly, they give range to the spine so it can bend and twist as required. Protecting the spine means protecting these all-important discs. And that is achieved by strengthening the back and by learning posture control.

>> **posture** and the back

Posture is important both to the strength of your back and to how you appear. It can make you look dumpy, tired, and old, or together, confident, and lithe. Fortunately, posture is not all down to your genetic inheritance. There is much you can do to improve it and prevent gravity from winning out.

The slump
This posture pushes the head forward out of line, rounds the shoulders, and leads to a slouched pelvis. Besides being esthetically unappealing, it places enormous strain on the discs.

The sway back
Runway models perform the sway to make themselves appear "cool." The sway back posture makes the shoulders lean and compresses the lower spine while reversing the thoracic area. In a nutshell—stand up straight!

Hyperlordosis
This is an exaggerated curve of the lumbar spine. It weakens the springboard effect provided by the lower back to the rest of the spine. It also shortens the stabilizing muscles of the pelvis. It's not only pregnant women and those with apple-body types who fall into this category. Athletic people tend to get tight hips that can throw them into this posture.

Below left to right The slump, the sway back, and hyperlordosis are three typical bad postures. Each will cause problems for the body sooner or later.

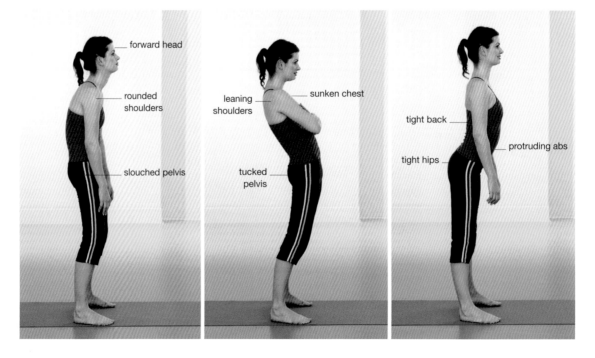

forward head
rounded shoulders
slouched pelvis

leaning shoulders
sunken chest
tucked pelvis

tight back
tight hips
protruding abs

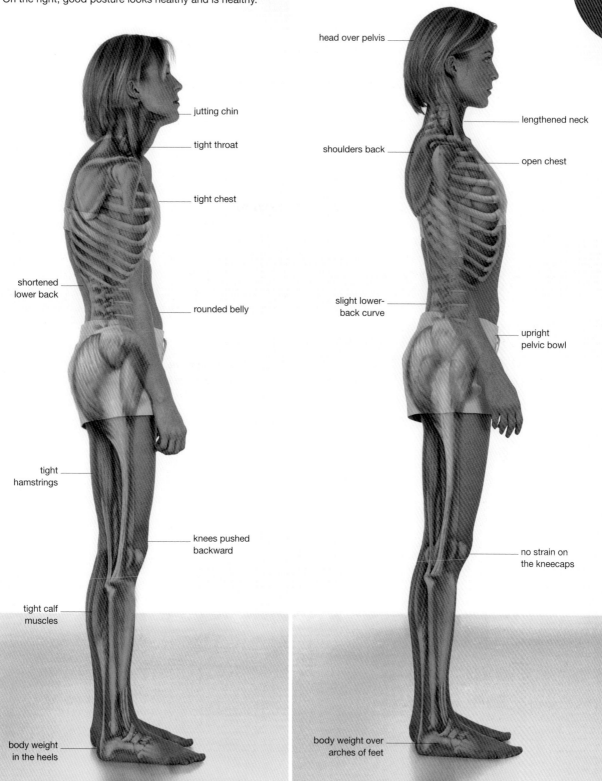

See the difference between bad and good posture. On the left, bad posture is sure to mean aches and pains. On the right, good posture looks healthy and is healthy.

head over pelvis

jutting chin

lengthened neck

tight throat

shoulders back

open chest

tight chest

shortened lower back

slight lower-back curve

rounded belly

upright pelvic bowl

tight hamstrings

knees pushed backward

no strain on the kneecaps

tight calf muscles

body weight in the heels

body weight over arches of feet

>> **protecting** the back

The back requires extra protection because it has so many interconnecting parts. If one part gets injured, so do all the others. There are certain moves we all perform every day that involve the back. Performing them correctly, as shown here, can go a long way in protecting the spine.

First position parallel means bringing your feet straight under your pelvis. It is the healthiest position to adopt for the legs and gives the greatest support for the spine.

"Butt-ski, out-ski" is the humorous name for this bending position (below right). It is ergonomically best for the discs of the lower back, which can be severely and irreparably damaged when bending, and particularly when lifting and twisting at the same time. It's really simple; just think of bending from the hips, sticking the bottom out, and using the legs to take the strain as you stand up.

The log roll is particularly helpful, especially for getting in and out of bed or up and down from lying on the floor. It's an excellent strategy when your back is painful and sore. It's shown on the opposite page in four simple steps.

Below left For first position parallel take the feet about 4 inches (10 cm) apart, with the second toe lining up with the kneecap and with the point midway on the groin line.

Below When you are bending, bend at the hips and keep the back straight. For lifting, always think "butt-ski, out-ski" (stick the bottom out) and lift with the legs.

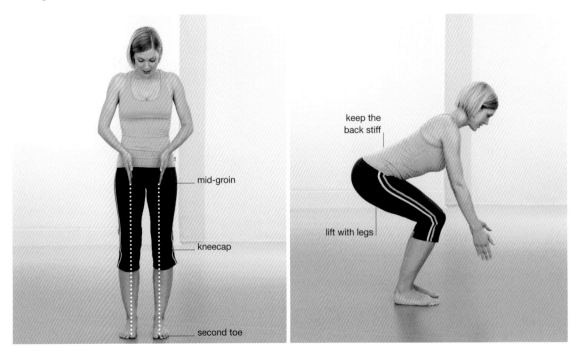

mid-groin

kneecap

second toe

keep the back stiff

lift with legs

log roll to get up safely

1 First, while lying on your back, tighten your waist and abdomen. Next, keep your back stiff just as in the "butt-ski, out-ski" position (see opposite) and brace your bent legs.

2 Roll onto your side as a unit with your shoulders and hips; don't twist at your waist. Keep your legs together. When getting out of bed, let your feet go over the side.

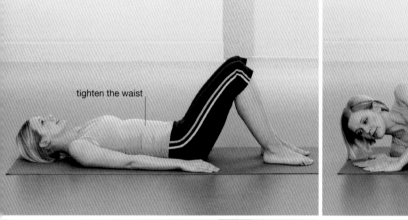

tighten the waist

keep the waist stiff

3 Next, use your arms, not your back, to push yourself up to sitting. When getting out of bed, let your feet dangle over the edge as soon as possible.

4 Sit tall, lift your breastbone and bring your head over the pelvis. Press down on your sitbones and straighten up through your spine. Feel as if your spine is being sucked up through a straw toward your head.

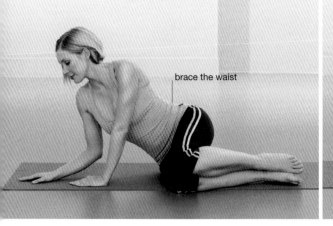

brace the waist

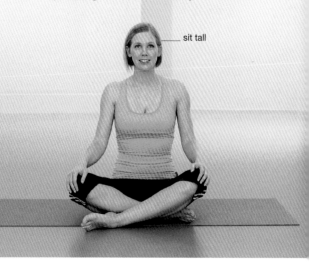

sit tall

>> **imagery** and cues

I like to use imagery and cues when I teach. They make all the difference to how you execute the movements and so will help you gain maximum benefit from the exercises. Here are some of the images demystified for you. Get to know them to bring more quality and greater detail to your movements.

The imagery I use is for you to hold in your mind when you are making a movement, just as an actor imagines and acts out a role during a performance. It is the same when someone is exercising. The phrases, or cues, guide the exerciser to know exactly how and when to execute the movement. You will quickly become familiar with the imagery and cues and you'll find that they promote the concentration and complexity needed to make your exercise more precise, and so most effective.

Follow the cues

Make smile lines These are two arc shapes that can be seen at the very tops of the legs when you tighten the hips and the backs of the thighs. They mark the separation of the muscles of the buttocks and the hamstrings.

Go into tabletop position is an image used to help you get your entire back, when you are on all fours, parallel to the floor. Your back should look just like the flat surface of a tabletop.

Imagine pressing pearls into sand is a term used to help you articulate each individual vertebra of the

Below left "Smile lines" delineate the buttocks from the hamstrings. **Center** "Pull the navel to the spine" tells you to bring the abs in firmly. **Below right** "Zip up the tight jeans" helps you to lift the abs.

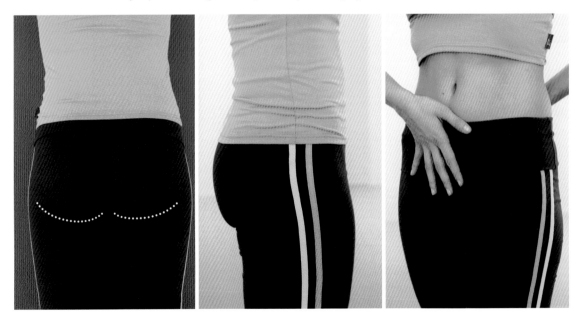

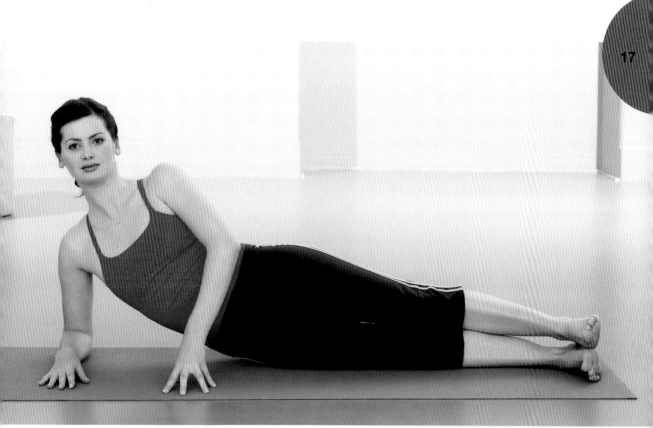

Above In this exercise, one of the keys to achieving a good pose is to feel the navel engaging to the spine—in other words, pulling the abdominal muscles firmly inward.

spine separately. When you are lying on your back, after lifting your pelvis off the floor, you lower the spine sequentially, one vertebra at a time, imagining as you do so that each vertebra is pressing a pearl, or bead, into soft sand beneath your body.

Take the head over the pelvis helps to ensure correct posture by eliminating slumping and a forward head.

Feel imaginary hands creating a sandwiching effect helps you to coordinate abdominal tension with back tension to give a stiffer, straighter trunk.

Imagine swimming-pool water is used when your abdomen is facing the floor to make you feel as if water is pressing upward against your abdomen. It helps you to lift the contents of your abdomen.

Lift the pelvis means to engage the muscles that stop the flow of urine and that stop you from breaking wind. Gently feel these muscles pull up toward your head, just as you would lift the arches of your feet to keep your ankles from wobbling.

Funnel the ribs helps you achieve a better upper-body crunch. First you "deflate" the breastbone, meaning that you compress it toward the ground. Then, as you start to curl your shoulders off the floor, you literally pull your ribs toward your pelvis, instead of just hinging at the waist.

Pull the navel to the spine means to pull the abdominals strongly inward.

Zip up the tight jeans means to lift the abdominals upward from the pubic bone toward the navel. It is the movement you need to zip up tight jeans.

Go into puppy-dog position means lying on your back with your legs and arms bent and off the floor. This allows you to engage your core muscles fully.

Imagine a dog's tail between the legs gives precision when you are doing pelvic tilts lying on your back. The image helps you curl your pelvis into a rounded shape as you imagine the connection between the fused vertebrae of your sacrum and the coccyx or very end of your spine.

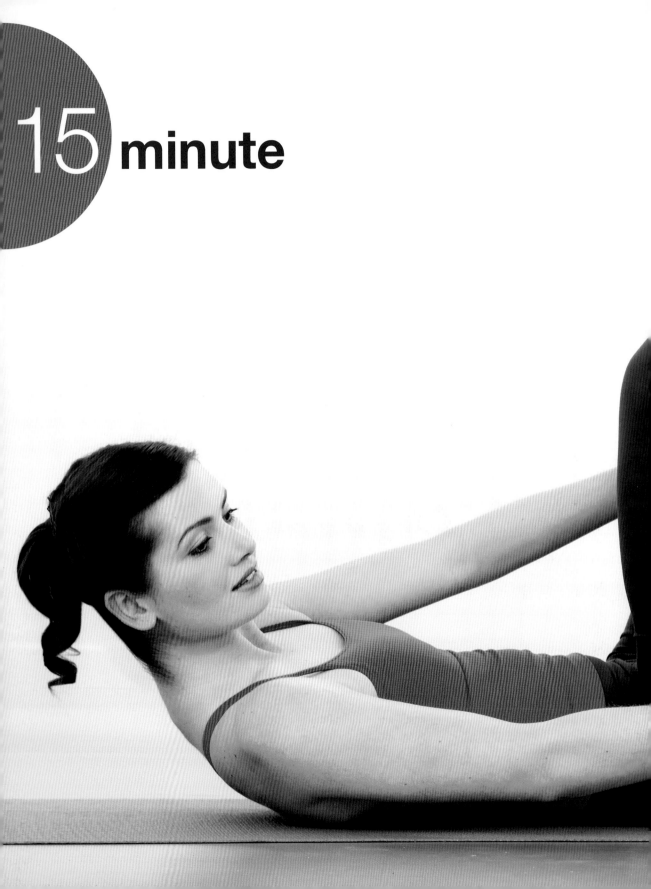

15 minute

Learn to make your
repetitions count.
Strive to feel what the
body is doing. Find
more in each exercise.

developing
the back >>

>> **developing** the back

Developing the back means making your back grow stronger with each exercise. Your mantra is to concentrate on making every repetition count. As you exercise, focus on the strength and beauty of your back. It is just as if you had planted a tree and were watching the trunk becoming stronger.

Because our bodies are highly efficient, they always take the path of least resistance. Making them work just that little bit harder can be difficult and requires discipline. This program sets the tone for the work that is to come. You learn to concentrate on the details so your body is encouraged to do more. Lengthen your body just a little bit more, bend even more deeply into your legs, reach your arms just a fraction higher. Perform each exercise and then next time go just a bit further with it. Be mindful that you can always do better. Stopping because you are not good enough is not an option. If you were perfect before you started any exercise, how would you derive satisfaction from your efforts? Fifty percent of success is simply showing up. The other 50 percent is working on and embellishing each exercise you do.

The exercises

Carry the feeling of elongating your body in the Body Yawn into the upright stance of the Knee Circles. Increase that feeling of length in the Side Stretch. The Squat Stretch may seem intimidating but it is excellent for gaining a sense of separating your trunk from your legs so that you can feel the length of your entire back. Modify the squat by not going too deeply. If your neck becomes too tight in the Toe Touches, keep your head down. Make yourself work in the Side Bends by not collapsing as you bend to the side, and maintain the tension top to bottom to keep the Overhead Squeeze intense. Plank exercises are always the most

> >> **tips for** developing the back
>
> - **Make your repetitions count** by paying attention to details throughout each exercise and by maintaining that attention.
>
> - **Register which body parts are moving,** and strive to feel the motion.
>
> - **Don't let the body** take the path of least resistance. Lose yourself in the details and try to find more in each exercise.
>
> - **Use modifications (see below),** as you exercise then, every time you repeat, you'll be pleasantly surprised to see that you are able to do a bit more.

difficult. If you need a place to begin, modify the Plank Push-up by lowering your knees to the floor for the duration of the exercise. Soon you'll notice that your shoulders will be able to bear more weight. Go further with the exercises you feel most comfortable with, but remember that it's normal to feel awkward with unfamiliar moves or to have mild soreness after the first try. Soon you'll feel as if you were made to exercise.

Developing the back takes time, patience, and discipline. Work diligently at the details and you will gradually manage to perform every exercise a little better than before.

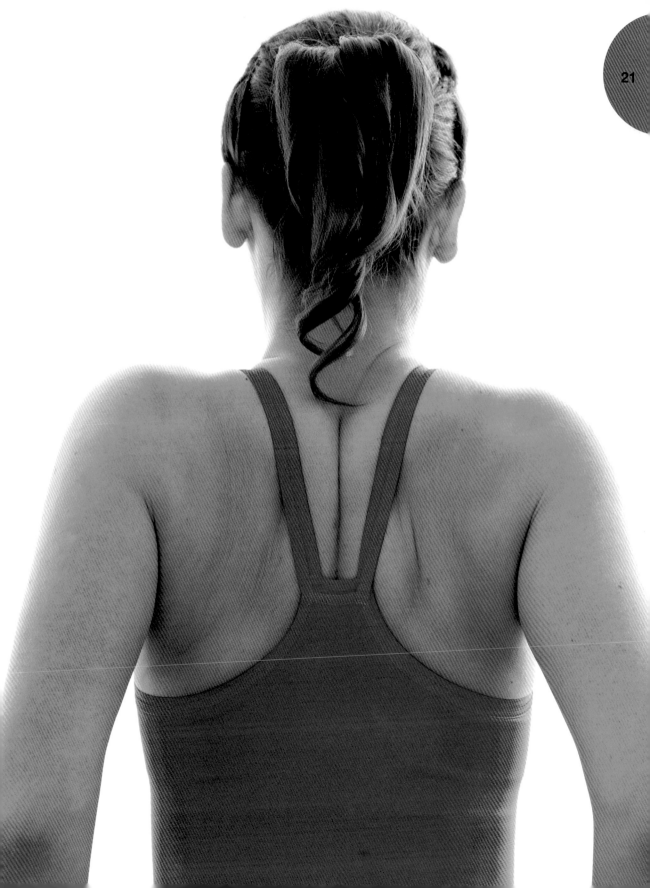

>> **limbering** upper rolls

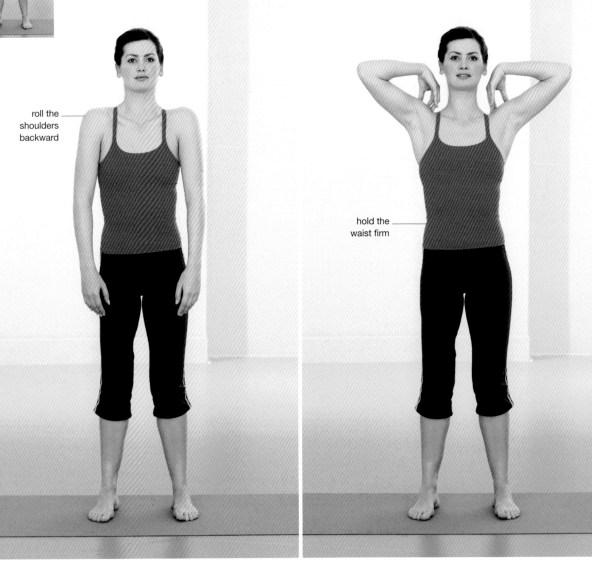

1 Stand tall with your feet about shoulder-width apart. Zip up the tight jeans (see p. 17) in the front and in the back. Open your chest and take your head over your pelvis (see p. 17). Breathe in and out as you count to 8 while slowly rolling your shoulders backward.

2 Hold your waist firm. Fold your elbows, and bring your hands to your shoulders. Make full, yet comfortable circles with your elbows about 5 times. Then reverse the direction for 5 more circles.

roll the shoulders backward

hold the waist firm

>> **elongating** body yawn

3 Place your feet just past shoulder-width apart. Reach your arms up sideways with your palms facing forward. Reach up and wide. Open your mouth and eyes.

4 Balance on your left leg, then exhale and squeeze your right knee to your waist. Find your balance, then return to stand on both feet with your arms reaching upward. Now balance on your right leg and squeeze your left knee to your waist. Repeat this alternation from right to left for 3 more sets.

reach up strongly

keep the hip firm

take feet just past shoulder-width

>> **stabilizing** knee circles

5 Stand on your left leg and be aware of your balance. Tighten your abdominals and hold your right knee steady to your waist with both hands. Anchor your shoulders back. Hold onto a piece of furniture if you can't manage to balance. Circle your knee 3 times.

6 Exhale and bow your head to your right knee and feel the stretch in your back. Release. Stand on your right leg and repeat the balance and circles. End with a bow to your left knee.

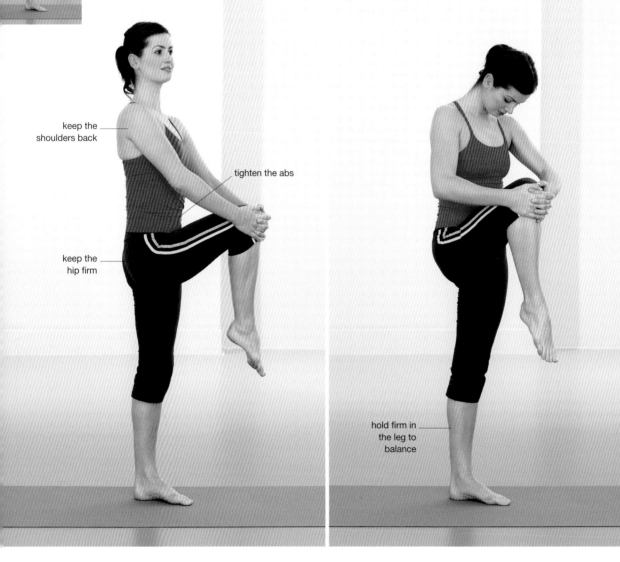

keep the shoulders back

tighten the abs

keep the hip firm

hold firm in the leg to balance

7 Stand and balance on your right leg. Cross your left foot over in front of your right ankle. Reach your right arm up and over your head toward the left.

reach up through the fingers

8 Zip up the tight jeans and firmly push the left hand in a horizontal motion against the left hip so you bend to the left. Breathe in and out 4 times. Come back to center. Uncross the leg and repeat to stretch the left side the same way.

feel it here

hold the abs

tuck the hip in

>> **opposing** squat stretch

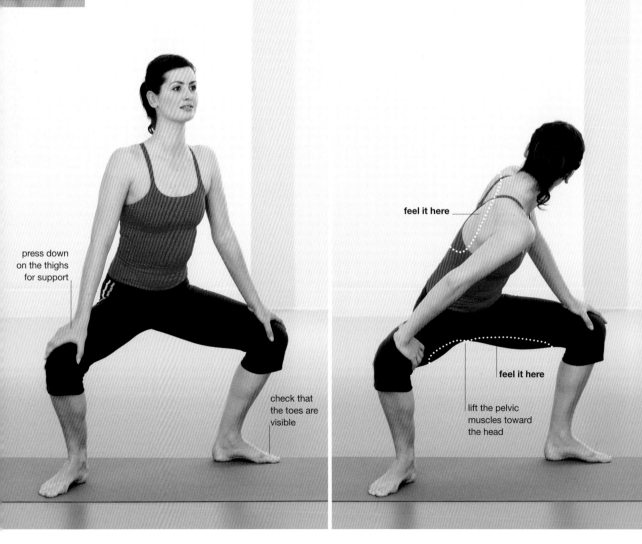

9 Open your legs past shoulder-width and turn your toes slightly outward. Hold your waist tight and firm your bottom as you bend straight down inside your legs to place your hands on top of your knees.

10 Lift your pelvis (see p. 17) and lengthen your spine. Inhale, press your right hand against your right knee, then exhale and turn your shoulders to look diagonally up and to your left. Breathe in and out 3 times. Stand up, then repeat the stretch to the other side.

press down on the thighs for support

check that the toes are visible

feel it here

feel it here

lift the pelvic muscles toward the head

>> **coordinating** toe touches

11 Lie down with your knees bent. Exhale, curl up your upper body, reach your hands out past your thighs, and take your feet off the floor. Look along your body. Take your left arm between your legs, reaching ahead with your middle fingers, and pull your head to your groin. Now lightly touch the toes of your left foot to the floor.

press the lower back into the floor

strongly reach the middle fingers out parallel to the floor

12 Simultaneously touch the right foot to the floor as you raise the left. Alternate toe touches for 16 repetitions. Place the right arm between the legs and alternate toe touches 16 more times. To end, hold both legs and arms up and increase the pull of the middle fingers.

intensify by reaching harder with the fingers

>> **articulating** side bends

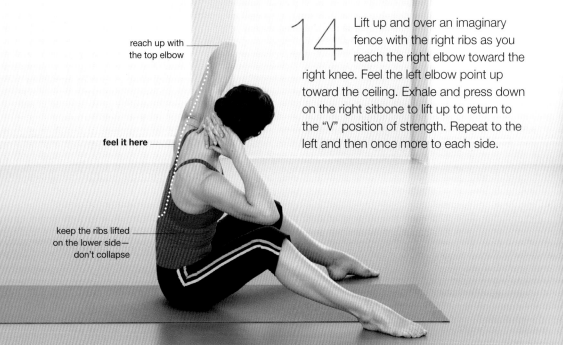

13 Sit on your sitbones with your legs shoulder-width apart and the soles of your feet on the floor. If you can't sit up straight, sit on a book or pillow. Line your head up directly over your pelvis. Place your hands behind your head and feel the "V" of strength running in a line from your lower back up and out of your elbows. Take your navel to your spine (see p. 17).

lift the skin of the
lower back upward

place soles of the
feet on the floor

14 Lift up and over an imaginary fence with the right ribs as you reach the right elbow toward the right knee. Feel the left elbow point up toward the ceiling. Exhale and press down on the right sitbone to lift up to return to the "V" position of strength. Repeat to the left and then once more to each side.

reach up with
the top elbow

feel it here

keep the ribs lifted
on the lower side—
don't collapse

>> **elongating** overhead squeeze

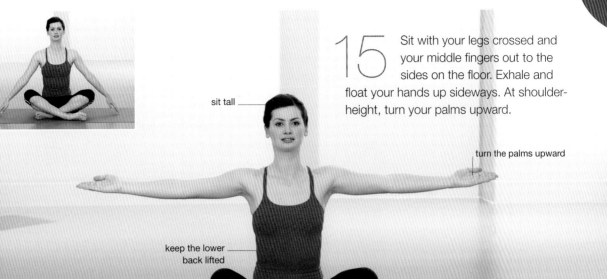

sit tall

turn the palms upward

keep the lower
back lifted

15 Sit with your legs crossed and your middle fingers out to the sides on the floor. Exhale and float your hands up sideways. At shoulder-height, turn your palms upward.

cross the thumbs
and press the little
fingers together

stay lifted

16 Continue reaching upward until the hands meet over the head. Cross the thumbs, press the palms together, and squeeze the upper arms against the head. Then exhale, sit taller, and open the arms back down. Keep the spine tall as you lower the arms sideways, turning the palms downward as you reach shoulder-height. Take the middle fingers to the floor. Repeat once more.

>> **accentuating** temple

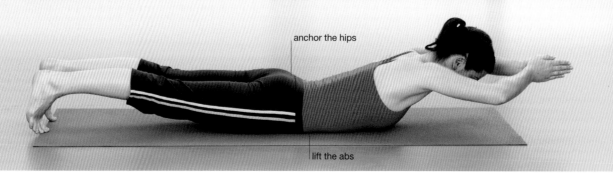

17 Lie on your front. Feel the imaginary swimming-pool water lift your abdominals off the floor (see p. 17). Reach your hands above your head on the floor, with elbows bent and palms together. Knit your ribs together to engage your solar plexus. Tuck your toes under to make little stands. Make smile lines (see p. 16).

pull the tailbone toward the heels

tuck the toes under

18 Inhale, then exhale as you levitate the hands and forearms off the floor, while at the same time straightening the knees so they come off the floor as well. Stay as you take a couple of breaths, then exhale and lower. Relax and then repeat the sequence.

anchor the hips

lift the abs

>> **stabilizing** oppositional lifts

19 Go onto all fours. Feel the swimming-pool water underneath the torso. Keep the elbows a little bent. Exhale and slide the second toe of the right foot behind you until the knee is straight, and at the same time slide the left middle finger out along the floor until the elbow is straight.

the toe barely
touches the floor

the fingers
barely
touch the
floor

20 Exhale and levitate the right foot and left hand up until they are horizontal. Stay and inhale, then exhale as you lower just to touch the fingertip and tops of the toes to the floor. Reach out and away from the torso to repeat. Breathe and lower. Repeat to the other side.

avoid any swing
of the hip

feel it here

feel it here

feel it here

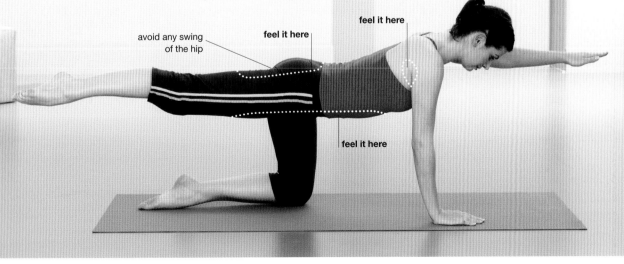

>> **powering** plank push-up

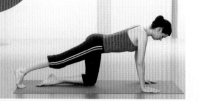

21 Go onto all fours. Feel the imaginary swimming-pool water up against the abdominals and hands sandwiching the lower back (see p. 17). Exhale and reach the right leg behind you and tuck the toes under to make a stand. Then exhale and reach the left leg behind you. This position is called a full plank.

tuck the toes under

22 Inhale, bend the elbows, and lower yourself in push-up style. Make smile lines. Exhale and stay, then inhale, exhale, and come back up. Feel as if your abdominals have lifted you. Break at one hip and then the other to return to all fours. Repeat once more.

hold the abs firm

developing the back >>

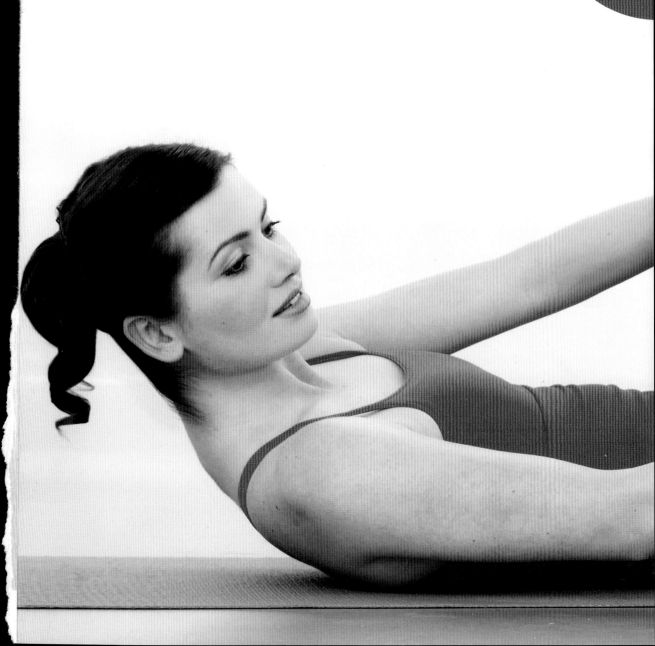

summary developing the back

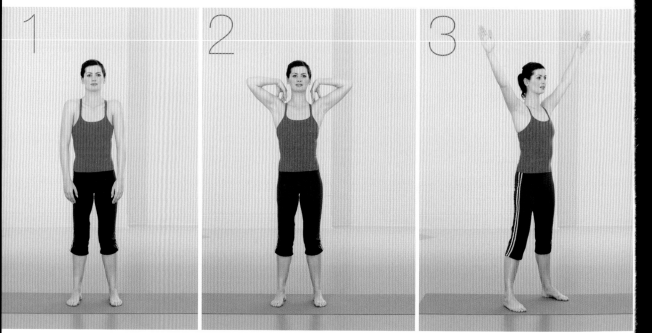

▲ **Limbering** Upper Rolls, page 22   ▲ **Limbering** Upper Rolls, page 22   ▲ **Elongating** Body Yawn, page 23

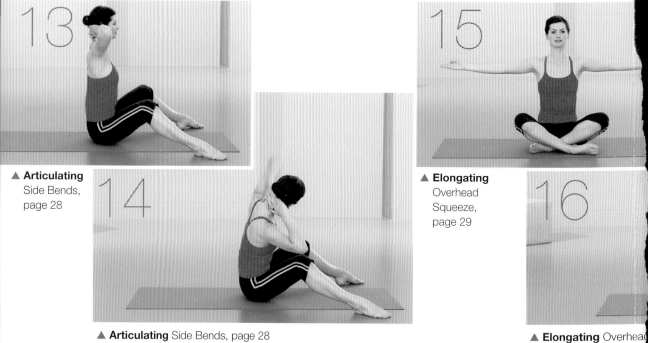

▲ **Articulating** Side Bends, page 28

▲ **Articulating** Side Bends, page 28

▲ **Elongating** Overhead Squeeze, page 29

▲ **Elongating** Overhead

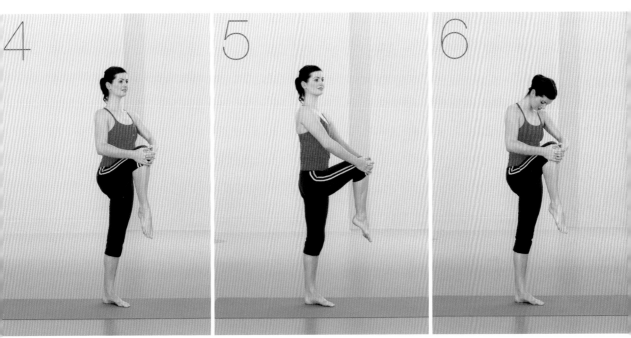

▲ **Elongating** Body Yawn, page 23   ▲ **Stabilizing** Knee Circles, page 24   ▲ **Stabilizing** Knee Circles, page 24

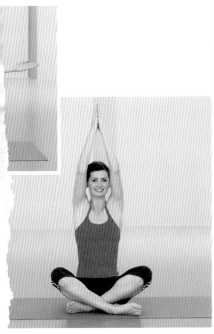

d Squeeze, page 29

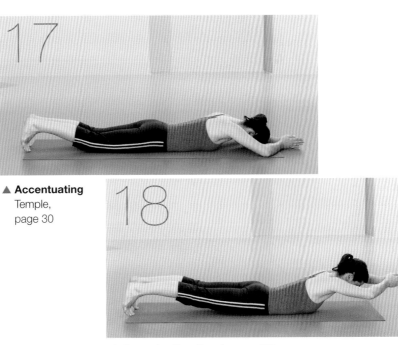

▲ **Accentuating**
Temple,
page 30

▲ **Accentuating** Temple, page 30

>> **centering** angel wings

23 Lie on your back. Feel the breath filling your torso as you inhale. Stretch your ankles away from your head. Lengthen your body. Exhale, then make angel wings with your arms, sliding your hands toward your hips as you bend your knees, raise your feet, and drag your feet toward your hips.

take the feet toward the hips

make angel wings with the arms

24 Reach to grab your heels, curling your body up into a little ball. Then inhale, lengthen your hips and legs down onto the floor again, and repeat 3 more times. Hold and intensify the last curl, tightening your abdominals, then relax to the floor.

curl up into a ball

15 minute **summary**

>> **developing the back** FAQs

Before you can develop your back, you have to learn to feel every part of it. Here are some tips to help you delve more deeply and attain the satisfaction of a well-developed upright back. Notice how others will start to comment on your new vertical posture, and may even give you compliments about your weight! An elongated back elongates the waist.

 Why is the **squat stretch** so important?

It helps you to find the bottom of the trunk. Everyone can easily feel the spine around the waistline, but most people need help in feeling what happens at the end of the pelvis. To develop the back, you have to find the entire length. At first the squat will seem as if it's only an inner-thigh stretch, but over time you'll be able to bend more deeply into the position and feel your buttocks moving toward the floor. The twist in the position opens the right and left sides of the back of the rib cage, helping you to open up the chronically stiff mid-back.

 Are the **toe touches** simply abdominal exercises or is there more to them than that?

While it does appear that the Toe Touches are all about the abdominals, they are working on other important features that help develop a strong back. They strengthen the deep hip flexors and train the legs to use the back more than the dominant thighs while you're standing and walking. When the thighs become more dominant than the back, the back gets weaker and makes you lean forward from the hips, giving you a bulky, bent-over appearance.

>> How do the **side bends** benefit the back?

They work specifically on both sides of the back. The great thing about the technique used for the Side Bends in this program is that it works not only the oblique abdominals but also the paraspinals—the long straplike muscles that run down each side of the back. The muscles tighten as they shorten but also tighten as they lengthen on the other side as you bend. Tightening as the muscles lengthen actually strengthens the back the most.

>> I feel my back caving in as I try the **oppositional lifts**. Is there any advice you can offer me?

The Oppositional Lifts may look simple, but they require special attention if you are to line up the back correctly. Mind all the cues before you move out of the preparatory position, since it's very easy for the back to go into the "old gray mare" position where the abdomen falls toward the floor once the limbs start to move. This is a sign of core weakness. The cue to feel the swimming-pool water underneath the abdomen always helps to lift the abdominals strongly up and away from the floor. So hold your core very strongly, and make sure you slowly slide the opposite hand and foot out before you perform the lifts.

>> I don't see how the **overhead squeeze** is developing my back if I'm not bending it. Help!

The Overhead Squeeze is a powerful exercise for developing the very deep postural muscles of the spine. It also helps us learn what a correct upright position is. Think of the back like an accordion. When the accordion is inflated with air, it's nice and elongated; when the air goes out, it deflates and the pleats become very prominent. This image is quite similar to the vertebral bones. The arms are very heavy and are culprits in promoting slumping (deflating the accordion) in the back. Attempting to sit as tall as we can, against the weight of the arms pulling us downward, is a very good exercise in sitting tall in general. I actually recommend you do the sit tall part, even without the arm lifts, a couple of times every day, at your computer, or in the car, for example. You'll be amazed at your improved posture!

>> I feel my back come off the floor when I do the **angel wings** exercise. Is that all right?

Often the back of the rib cage is very tight, and people are not able to get the back of the waist and the back of the rib cage on the floor at the same time. A great goal to progress toward with this exercise would be eventually to be able to stabilize your back enough to get its entire length—the rib cage, the waist and the pelvis—against the floor. If you persist for two months, you'll probably attain your goal. Be sure to do the final step of the exercise, where you hold onto your heels, or your legs, while you pull your shoulders toward the knees. That will help you to stretch the parts of the back you need in order to lie flat with the whole back on the floor.

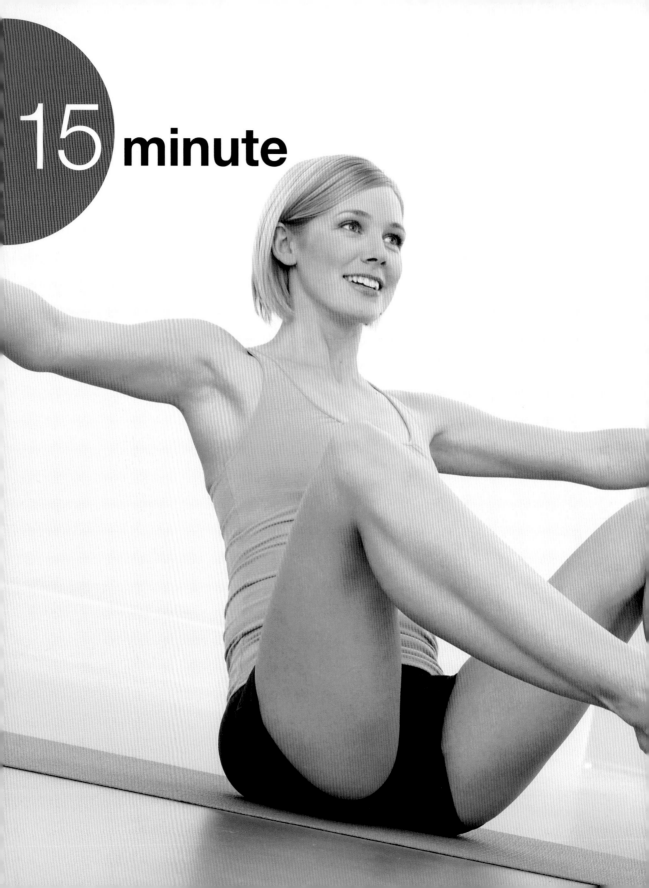

15 minute

Accentuate the
changing rhythms.
Notice your breath.
Oxygen is key.

revitalizing
the back >>

>> **revitalizing** the back

We are all living longer lives and we all want to live in the best of health. Regularly revitalizing and renewing the cells of the body by eating well and staying mobile is key. Working on revitalizing the back is one of the cornerstones of health. It enables us to remain active for as long as possible.

Revitalizing literally means to restore life, to bring vitality. Our breath is what revitalizes us. The lungs hold a potential for an abundance of oxygen. In this series we vary breath patterns in order to manifest this abundance. This variety of patterns is accomplished by virtue of the exercises' different rhythms and cadences. Although the exercises will guide your breath, remember to use the general breath pattern of inhaling through the nose and exhaling softly out through the mouth. Don't inhale so strongly that the nostrils are forced together. Instead, be sure to keep them open and allow the air to flow toward the back of the nasal cavity, as if you were inhaling fine perfume. When you exhale, almost try to make a "ha" sound.

The exercises

This revitalizing program uses many quick repetitions to stimulate the body from different angles. The structure of the exercises forms the basis of the rhythms, which will regulate your breath as you exercise. Notice how the Arm Swing and the Leg Swing both have a waltzlike quality. The Tread in Place exercise has a marching rhythm. The Leg Circles are brisk and intense.

In the Tapping Chest exercise, you actually need to vocalize the exhalation each time. The sustained quality of the "O" Balance requires its own soft internal flow.

This program also includes the more difficult Prone Rocker and one of the hardest plank exercises—the Plank Balance. Both generate

> **>> tips for** revitalizing the back
>
> - **Each exercise has a natural rhythm.** As you exercise, accentuate this rhythm, as if you were showing a friend how to do it.
>
> - **Notice how your breath** subtly changes from exercise to exercise. Let your body go with the rhythm. Sometimes it even helps to hum along as you go.
>
> - **Inhale through the nose.** Direct the air into the back of the throat. Open the lips and gently exhale through the mouth.
>
> - **Modify when needed.** You can hold the Prone Rocker position still and simply hold the Plank Balance for a couple of breaths.

internal heat and will stoke the fire of revitalization within you. However, remember only to do as much as you are able without undue straining, or at worst, by holding your breath. If the Prone Rocker is difficult when you first try it, you can modify it by simply holding your hands and feet off the floor and eliminating the rock. For the Plank Balance, modify the exercise by remaining in a simple plank position, without lifting the foot.

Now take a deep breath and revitalize your body with these exercises. It's just like opening the window and breathing in fresh air.

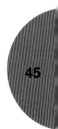

Open your lungs and breathe deeply in this revitalizing back workout. To get the best effect, pay attention to the rhythms and cadences of the exercises.

>> **opening** arm swing

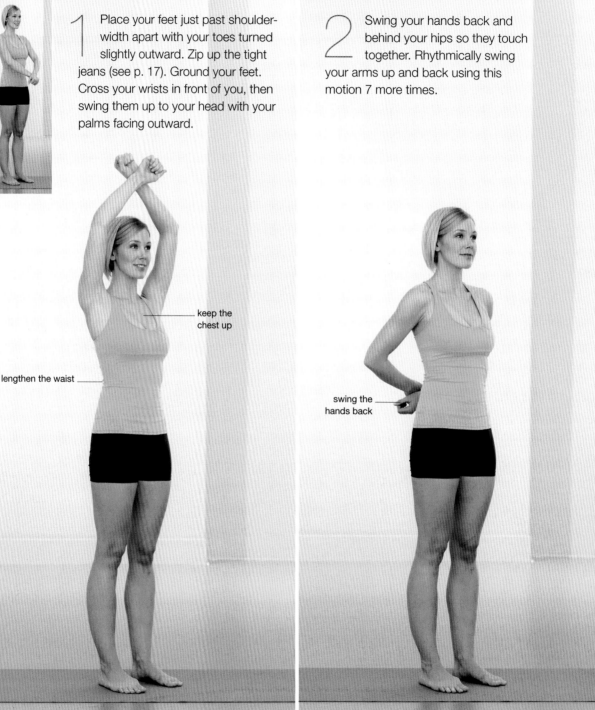

1 Place your feet just past shoulder-width apart with your toes turned slightly outward. Zip up the tight jeans (see p. 17). Ground your feet. Cross your wrists in front of you, then swing them up to your head with your palms facing outward.

2 Swing your hands back and behind your hips so they touch together. Rhythmically swing your arms up and back using this motion 7 more times.

keep the chest up

lengthen the waist

swing the hands back

>> **balancing** leg swing

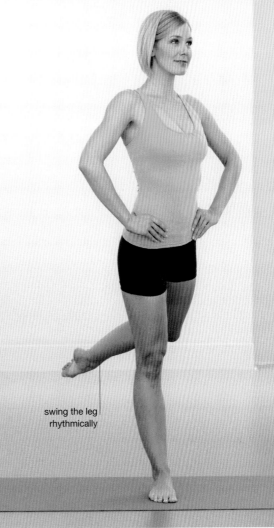

3   Stand tall with your hands on your hips. Balance on your right leg, using a hand on a piece of furniture to support you if you need. Hold your hip firm on your right leg. Keep your chest up. Swing your left foot in front, as if you were wiping your foot on the ground.

4   Then swing the left foot down and back. Repeat this forward and backward motion easily and rhythmically 7 more times. Find your balance on the left leg and repeat, swinging the right leg.

hold the hip firm
on the balance leg

swing the leg
rhythmically

>> **stimulating** tread in place

5 Stand tall with the feet just less than hip-width apart, hands on the hips. Take the head back over the pelvis (see p. 17). Pull the navel to the spine (see p. 17). Lift the abdominal area from the pubis to the navel. Let this lift help you rise up onto the balls of the feet.

6 Reach your head upward as you lower your right heel, then rise up on the balls of your feet and lower your left heel. Repeat this treading motion 32 times.

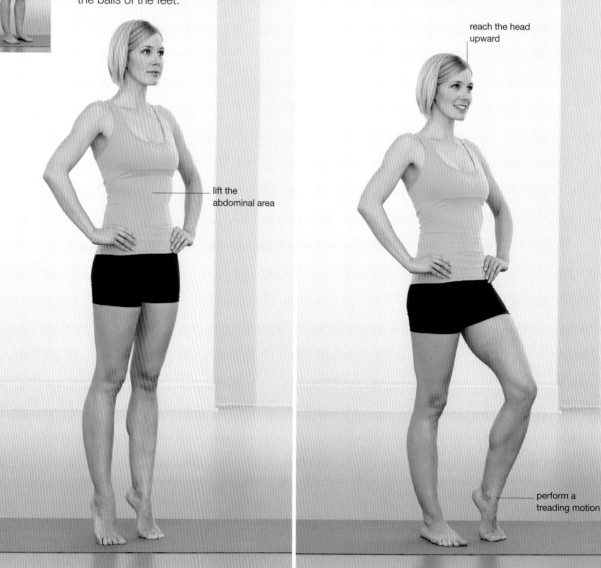

reach the head upward

lift the abdominal area

perform a treading motion

>> **opening** tapping chest

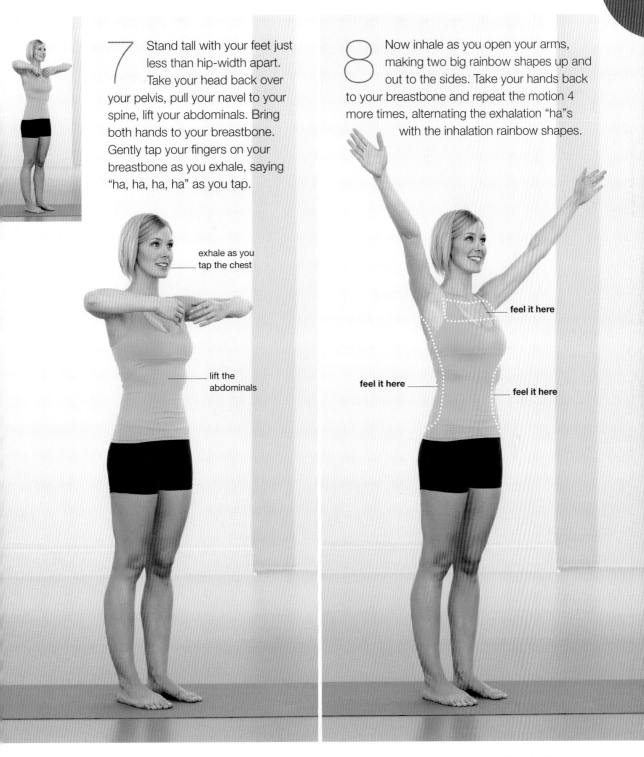

7 Stand tall with your feet just less than hip-width apart. Take your head back over your pelvis, pull your navel to your spine, lift your abdominals. Bring both hands to your breastbone. Gently tap your fingers on your breastbone as you exhale, saying "ha, ha, ha, ha" as you tap.

8 Now inhale as you open your arms, making two big rainbow shapes up and out to the sides. Take your hands back to your breastbone and repeat the motion 4 more times, alternating the exhalation "ha"s with the inhalation rainbow shapes.

exhale as you tap the chest

lift the abdominals

feel it here

feel it here

feel it here

>> **lengthening** side stretch 2

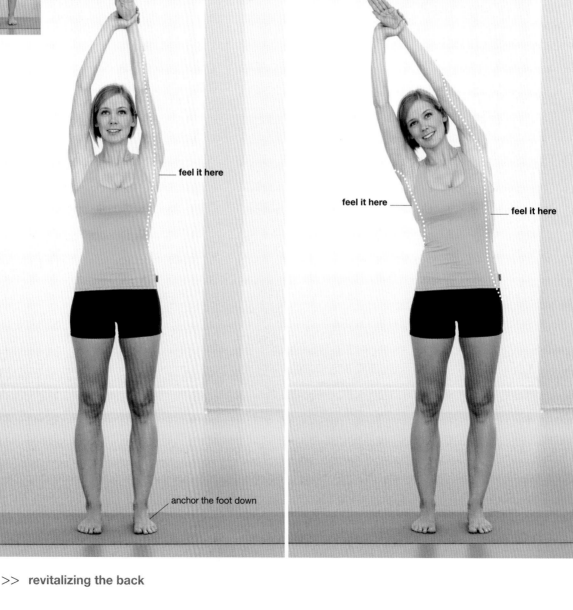

9 Stand with your arms above your head, and your feet about hip-width apart. Anchor your left foot downward as you grasp your left wrist with your right hand. Elongate and pull your wrist upward.

10 Inhale as you lift up, to the right, as though you were leaning over a fence. Stay, exhale, lengthen. Then inhale, stay, then exhale and anchor the left foot again as you stretch back up to vertical, lengthening the waistline. Take the arms down. Repeat to the other side.

feel it here

feel it here

feel it here

anchor the foot down

>> **revitalizing the back**

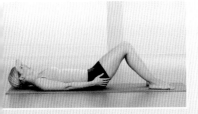

11 Lie on your back and bend your knees. Open your feet about shoulder-width apart. Place your left hand behind your head and hold behind your right thigh with your right hand. Exhale, deflate your breastbone, and funnel your ribs (see p. 17) toward the pelvis to curl up your upper body. Use your left arm to pull up higher.

hold the abs
firmly in

press the lower back
against the floor

12 Now stroke the right thigh from bottom to top with the right hand, as if you were stroking a cat. Reach out past the knee with the middle finger. Stroke 6 times, then intensify the last stroke. Lower the upper body to the floor, then change arms to repeat, using the left hand and stroking the left thigh 6 times.

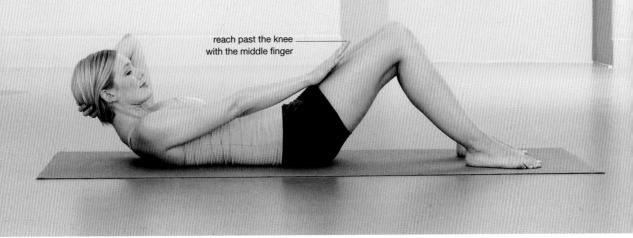

reach past the knee
with the middle finger

>> **coordinating** leg circles

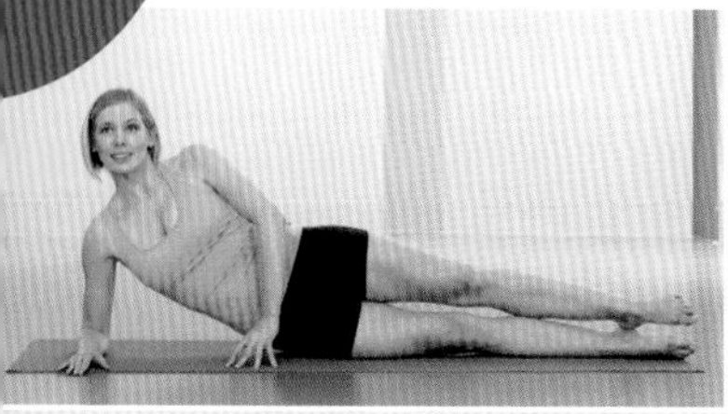

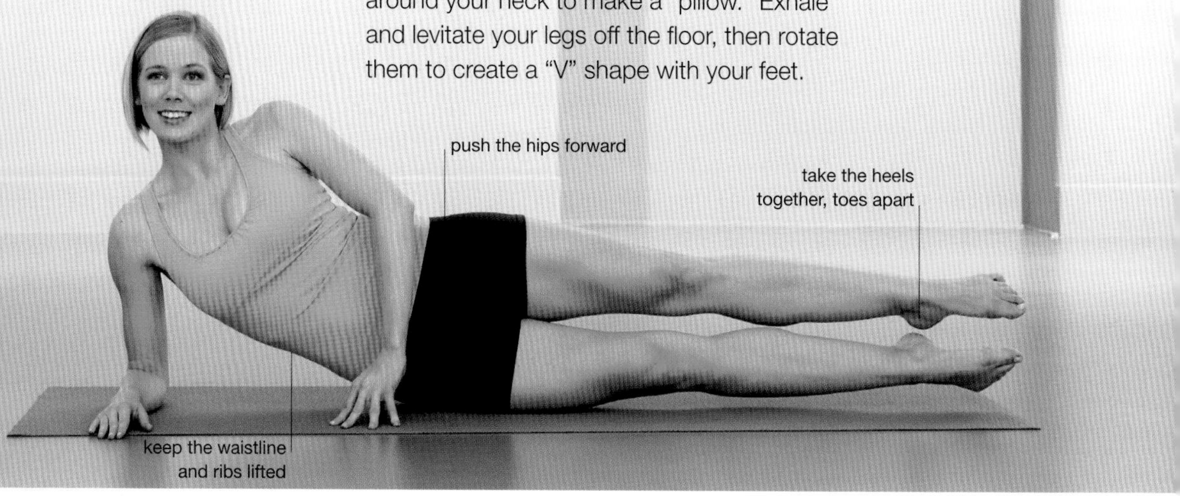

13 Lie on your right side in a straight line. Prop yourself up on your right forearm, using your left hand for balance. If you can't do this, lie on your shoulder with your arm folded and your hand around your neck to make a "pillow." Exhale and levitate your legs off the floor, then rotate them to create a "V" shape with your feet.

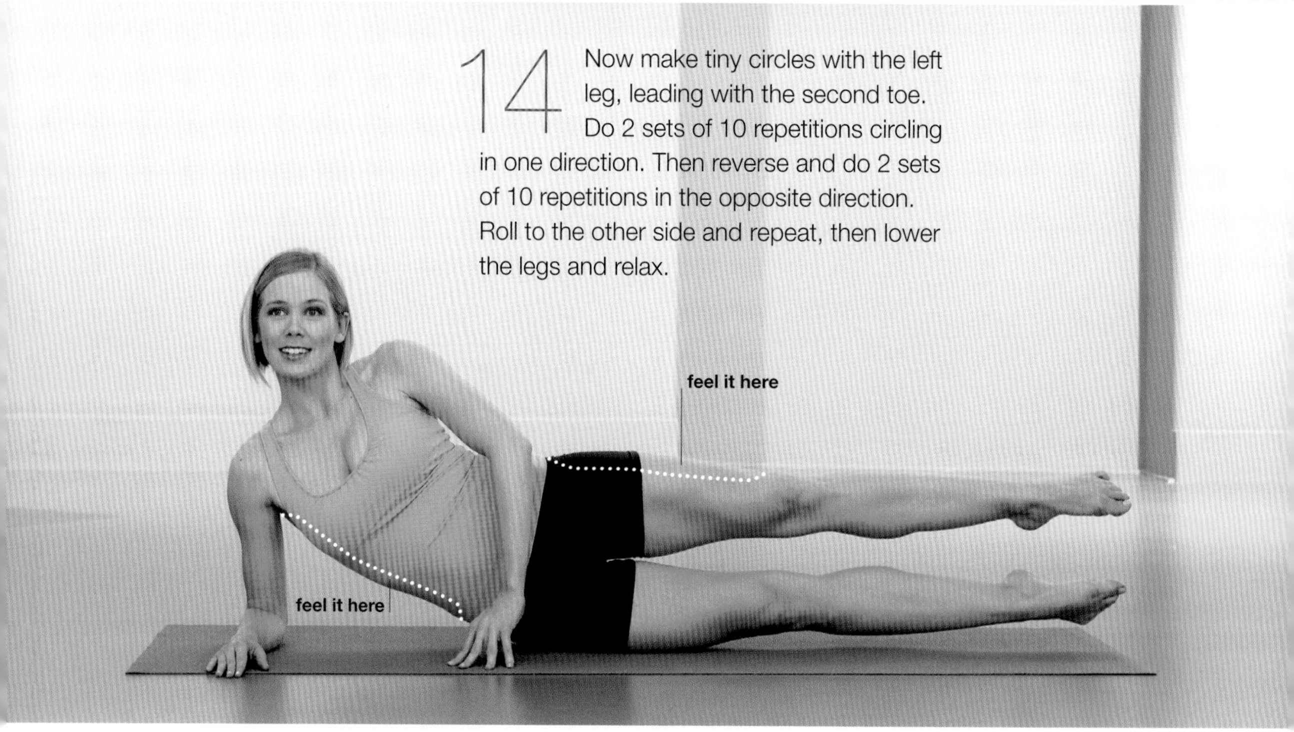

push the hips forward

take the heels together, toes apart

keep the waistline and ribs lifted

14 Now make tiny circles with the left leg, leading with the second toe. Do 2 sets of 10 repetitions circling in one direction. Then reverse and do 2 sets of 10 repetitions in the opposite direction. Roll to the other side and repeat, then lower the legs and relax.

feel it here

feel it here

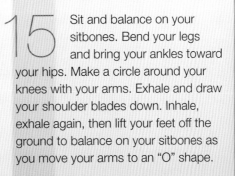

15 Sit and balance on your sitbones. Bend your legs and bring your ankles toward your hips. Make a circle around your knees with your arms. Exhale and draw your shoulder blades down. Inhale, exhale again, then lift your feet off the ground to balance on your sitbones as you move your arms to an "O" shape.

balance on the sitbones

16 Stay, feeling yourself getting taller, then exhale, press the hips down to the floor, open the arms, and take the arms back down to the knees. Repeat 2 more times.

lift the lower back

>> **accentuating** prone rocker

17 Lie on the front of your body. Reach your hands above your head on the floor about shoulder-width apart, palms face down. Exhale and drag your hands toward your upper chest to make the sphinx pose (left). Exhale, and levitate your feet off the floor about 2 inches (5 cm). Reach your hands in front of you to rock forward. Your legs will elevate as you go.

pull the tailbone
toward the heels

lift the abs

18 Lift up your head and push back up to catch yourself on your hands. Your legs will descend. Rock forward and back for 5 more repetitions. Hold the last position to stabilize your body, then relax.

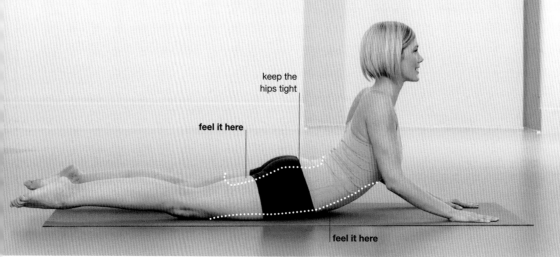

keep the
hips tight

feel it here

feel it here

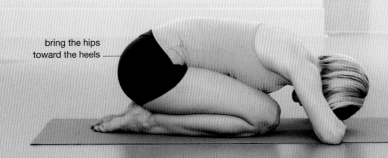

19 Kneel on the floor and bend forward, stretching your arms along the floor above your head. Push back, allow your knees to open a little, then bring your hips back toward your heels. Place your palms one on top of the other underneath your forehead.

bring the hips toward the heels

20 Inhale, push down on the hands, curl the head down, and round the back under, breathing in for 3 counts. Allow the hips to lift away from the feet a little. Bow the head and look toward the navel. Then exhale and lower the head and hips back toward the floor. Take 3 more in- and out-breaths as you perform this lifting and lowering motion.

let the hips lift

>> **powering** plank balance

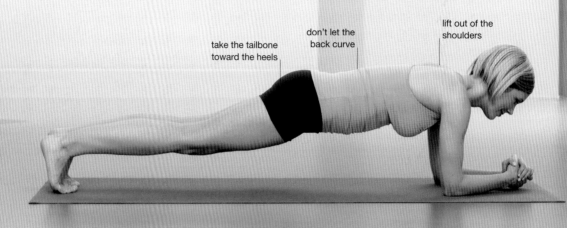

21 Go onto your forearms and knees, holding your hands together. Feel imaginary hands sandwiching your lower back (see p. 17). Exhale and reach your right foot behind you until your knee is straight, then reach your left foot behind you. Tuck your toes under to form 2 little stands. This is a forearm plank.

take the tailbone toward the heels

don't let the back curve

lift out of the shoulders

22 Exhale and balance on the left leg, pointing the toes of the right foot to the wall behind you. Breathe, then bring the right toes back under to the forearm plank position. Repeat to the other side, balancing on the right leg, then repeat to both sides once more.

lifts the abs

>> **centering** "C" exercise

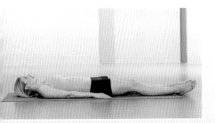

23 Lie on your back. Inhale, reach your arms up above your head on the floor, and clasp your hands. Stretch your ankles away from your head at the same time.

stretch the ankles away from the head

24 Slowly and smoothly slide your arms and legs to the right to make the letter "C" as seen from above. Repeat the body slide to the left. Feel as if your waist is lifting up and over an imaginary fence. Lengthen your body out, then repeat to the other side. Repeat another 4 times to right and left.

press the back onto the floor

revitalizing the back >>

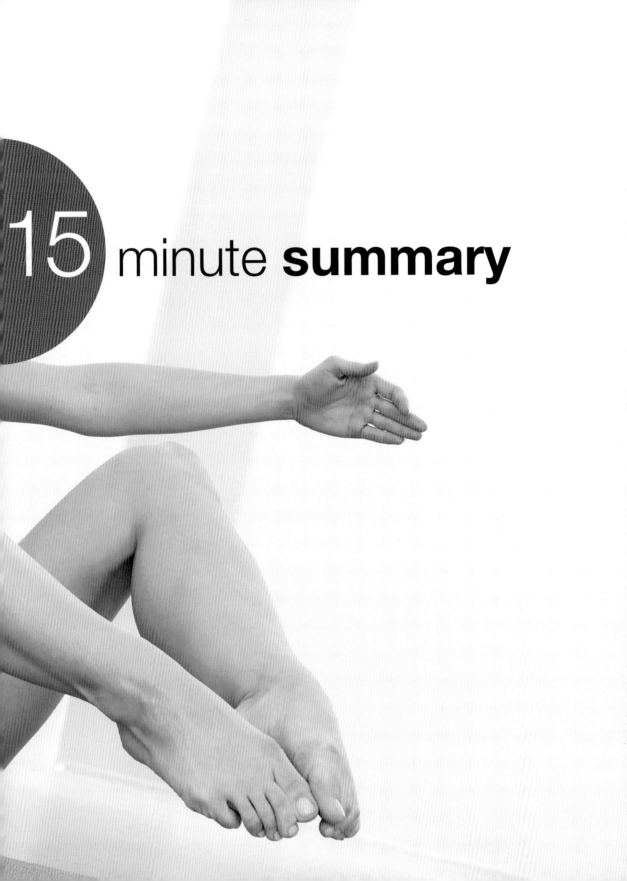

15 minute **summary**

>> **revitalizing the back** FAQs

Revitalizing the Back concentrates on the breath, and on oxygenating the body and the back. There are subtle modulations in our breath. These modulations may be imperceptible to others, but they can add a powerful element to your exercise. Learn to focus on them while you exercise and create a deeper, lasting effect for a stronger back!

>> I don't see how the **arm swings** and **leg swings** help with my breathing. Can you explain?

Simply lifting and lowering the arms forces the air in and out of the lungs and produces a ripple effect in the vertebrae of the mid- and upper back. To prove it, place your fingers on your upper back just below your neck at your shoulder line. Move the other arm up and down. You'll feel the subtle muscle activity. The pendulumlike leg swings cause muscle activity around the vertebrae of the lower back and pelvis, and force the breath to alter.

>> Can you explain why and how hard I have to tap the chest in the **tapping chest** exercise?

Tapping on the chest stimulates the lungs and heart. It also gives a light mobilization to the little joints between the breastbone and the ribs. When you loosen the breastbone joints, you also loosen the upper and mid-back since the ribs connect the two. I like to tap hard enough to make a hollow sound, which might take some practice. Only go as hard as your comfort level allows; the taps are taps, not large thumps. They should not cause bruising.

>> Why would **stroke the cat** revitalize me?

It does so thanks to a domino effect. It's a great way to round the back fully and this helps you work the upper abdominals. That promotes the opening of the mid- and upper back, which in turn opens the diaphragm—the main muscle that we use for breathing. A tight mid- and upper back prevents the back part of the diaphragm from working properly, so some of our potential oxygen supply is cut off.

>> Doesn't the **prone rocker** stop my breath? How do I not hold my breath in this exercise?

It's always a challenge and takes some practice to master breathing while lying on the abdomen. Then adding the lift of the abdominals, the pulling of the tailbone to the heels, and making smile lines at the tops of the thighs can be overwhelming. Remember that performance varies and every attempt will be a little different. First, line up the body before you begin to rock. When you rock forward, it will actually be natural to exhale through your mouth. Think of the inhalation as lifting you up before you catch yourself on your hands. It's often simplest just to exhale on the rock forward and you will then automatically inhale as you lift your shoulders up again.

>> I have bad knees. How can I do the **rest breather** other than on my knees?

One way to modify this exercise is to stay high in the all fours position, with the hands under the shoulders and the knees under the hips. Then it's more like the Cat and Camel exercise in the Soothing the Back program. Another modification is to lie on your side, hold onto your knees and breathe into your back. Yet another modification is to lie on your back, onto your knees and gently circle them, as in the Sacral Circles exercise of the Soothing the Back program.

>> I don't understand how the **plank balance** helps revitalize me, or how it uses my breath.

The Plank Balance, one of the hardest of the plank exercises, challenges the breath and increases body temperature because of its intensity. You have to breathe harder simply to maintain this position at all. Like the other programs, Revitalizing the Back is designed to help you be successful when you reach the hardest exercises. Those leading up to this one will have promoted greater use of the breathing muscles so that by the time you get to the Plank Balance, you have the best chance of achieving it. If you need to modify the exercise, especially if you find you are holding your breath, do so by staying with both feet on the ground. Another modification is to lower the knees to the ground, and hold yourself up with your forearms, knees, and toes.

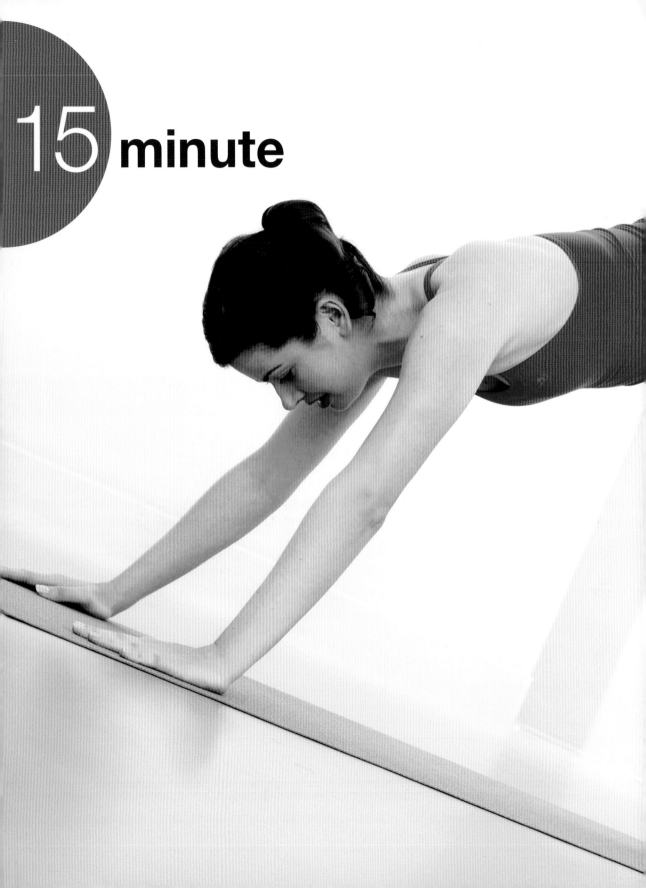

15 minute

energizing
the back >>

Work all parts of your back. Look for the sensitivity. Enjoy better whole-body movement.

>> **energizing** the back

Energizing the back can be misunderstood. It does not mean overusing or abusing the back. The spine is the all-important central command post for all movement. Here we activate it fully, as if each muscle cell were plugged into an electrical cord. The worthwhile result will be better whole-body movement.

The best way to energize the back is to activate and recruit the muscles fully—to turn the electricity on, and then turn up the volume. We do this by coordinating the breath with exercises that work the core—the deep abdominal muscles, the deep lower-back muscles; and the deep pelvic muscles. Do this series when you want a challenge. Persevere even if you have to modify the exercises or have to work up to doing all the repetitions. Staying with this program is important for beginners because it will fast-track your understanding of the muscles that need to work for your back to improve. But this program does not only contain essential core exercises. It also works the legs, which connect to and work with the core muscles. The result is an integrated, whole-body experience.

The exercises

Circling motions of the arms, hips, wrists, and ankles prime and energize the body for the later, more intense muscle-contracting exercises. The Hip Lift and Swimming exercises are among the greatest back-strengthening exercises. To modify the Hip Lift, open the legs and press down on the feet as you lift the hips. Pressing down on the feet and forearm, especially sideways, puts extra pressure on the bones. Our bones are only as strong as the pressure we apply to them. Space travel has proven the deleterious effect on bone density when atmospheric pressure is removed. So build up to this exercise, and you won't regret it when you take a tumble.

> ## >> **tips for** energizing the back
>
> - **Feel your back sensations increase.** Check to see if you can feel and identify all the parts of your back.
>
> - **Consciously breathe** through the intense parts of the exercises.
>
> - **Strive to make** your right side feel as sensitive as your left during this program.
>
> - **Imagine the electrical cord** connection between your conscious thoughts and the motions you make in each exercise. This will increase your mind–body connection, and fully energize your back.

Moving on through the program, the Swimming exercise creates endurance. If your back starts to tighten up, come down, breathe and relax, and then start again. The Compressions exercise, though less obviously intense, generates thorough use of the front of the body and activates the core. And for alignment and coordination of the core, the back, and the inner thighs—our "second spine"—work on First Position Abs and Puppy Dog Abs.

In an energized back the muscles work actively and powerfully with those of the core and the legs to ensure good whole-body movement.

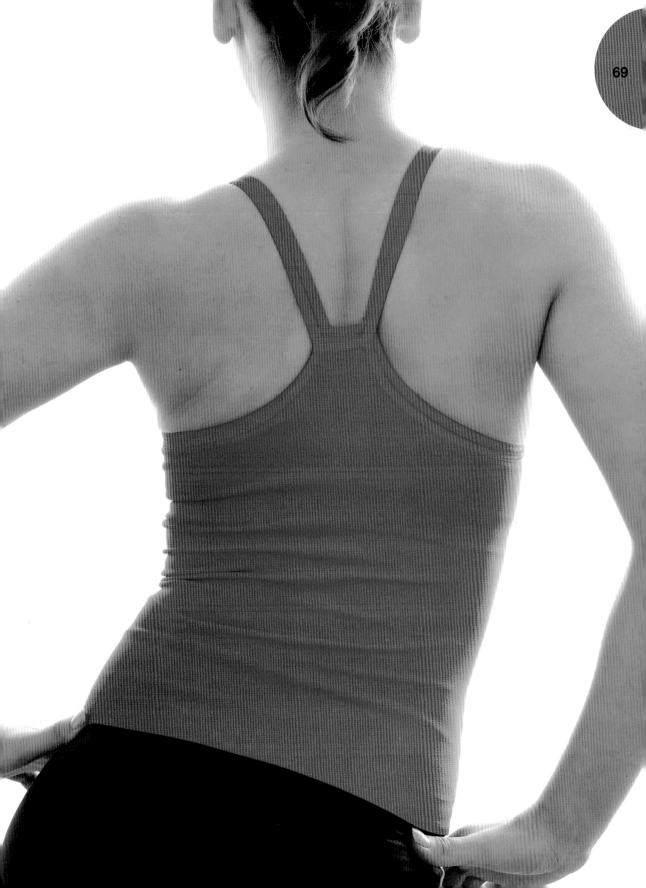

>> **limbering** arm circles

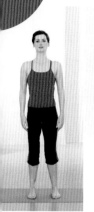

1 Stand with your legs shoulder-width apart. Reach both arms up overhead, and clasp your fingers. Lengthen your tailbone toward the ground. Circle your arms, imagining making 4 circles on the ceiling with your hands. Return to center.

2 Again, lift up and out of the waist and tighten the waist. Lengthen the tailbone. Reverse the movement with the hands, imagining making 4 more circles on the ceiling. Bring the arms down.

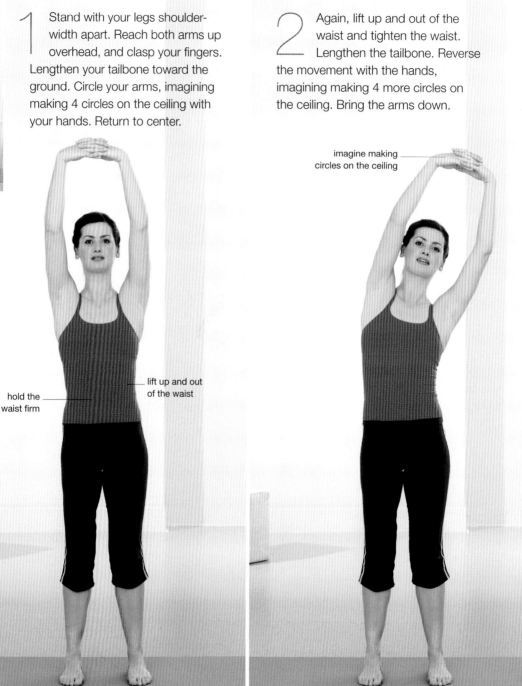

imagine making circles on the ceiling

hold the waist firm

lift up and out of the waist

>> **limbering** hip circles

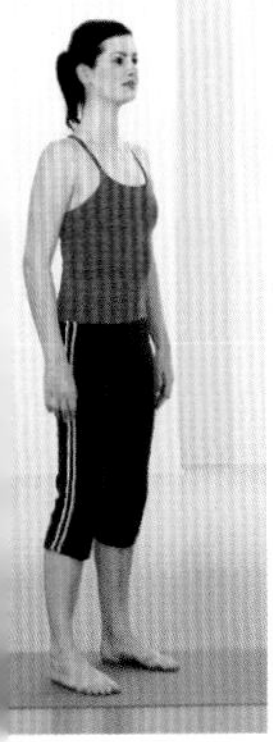

3 Stand with your legs about shoulder-width apart. Place your hands on your hips. Start moving your hips in a circling motion. Notice that your knees will also circle at the same time. Keep them a little bent. Be sure to tighten your waist. Circle your hips one way 5 times.

4 Still keeping the knees bent and the waist tight, circle the hips the other way 5 times. Repeat the hip circles again 5 times in each direction.

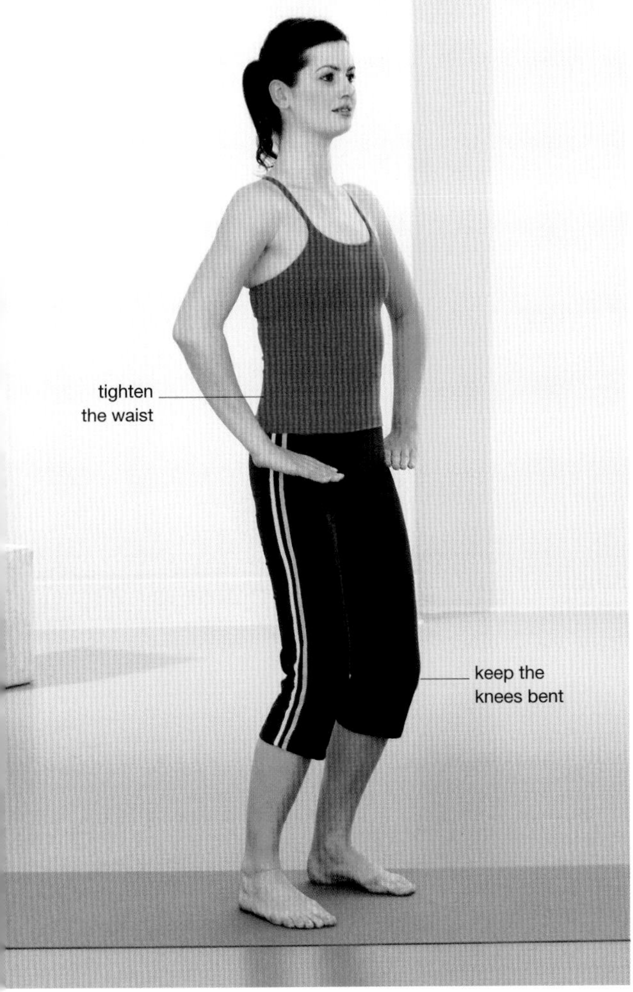

tighten the waist

keep the knees bent

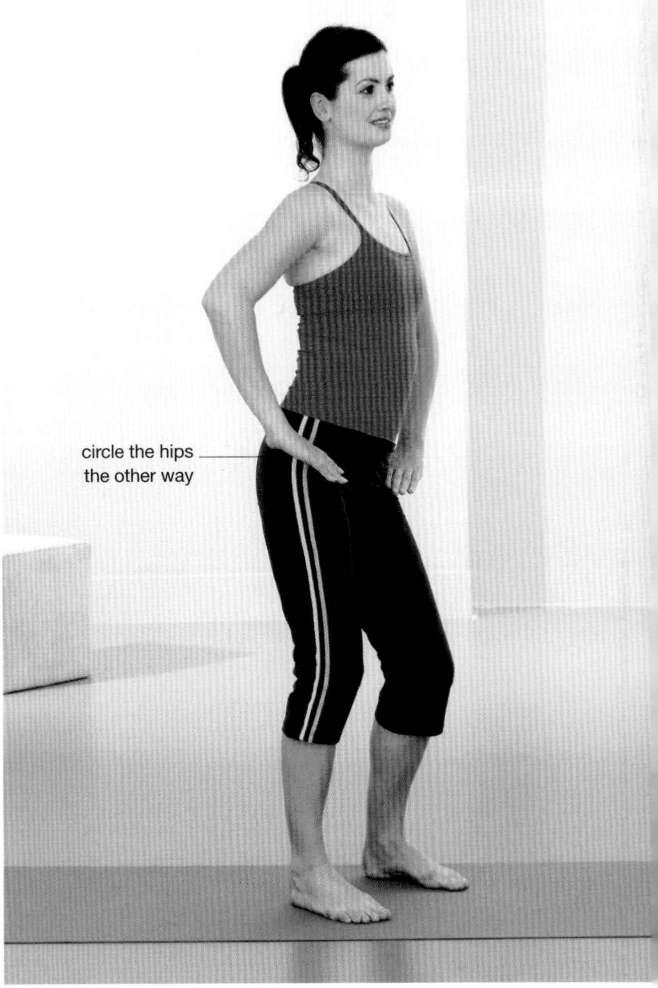

circle the hips the other way

>> **stabilizing** wrist and ankle circles

5 Stand with your legs about shoulder-width apart. Place your left hand on your left hip joint. Slowly shift onto your left leg, raise your right, and find your balance. Tighten in your waist to help with the balance or hold onto a chair. Press your left foot into the ground.

6 Circle the right ankle and right wrist at the same time. Circle 5 times. Reverse the direction for 5 circles. Repeat the whole exercise again, then shift onto the right leg and repeat, circling with the left foot and left hand. Take the left leg down to the floor.

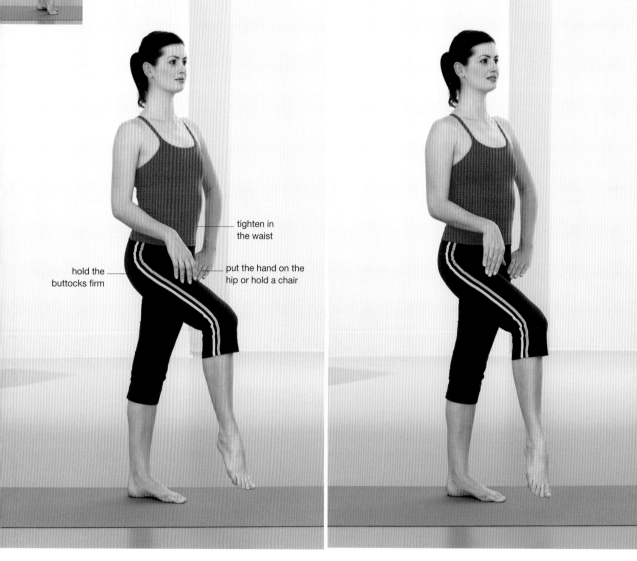

tighten in the waist

hold the buttocks firm

put the hand on the hip or hold a chair

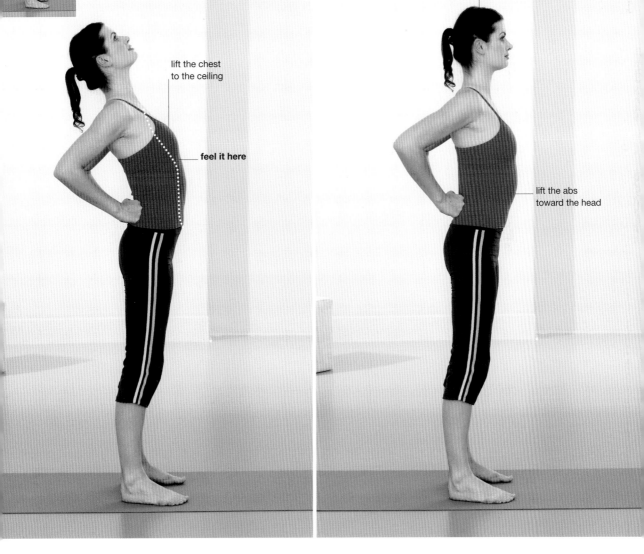

7 Stand tall with your feet just less than hip-width apart. Take your head over your pelvis (see p. 17). Pull your navel to your spine (see p. 17). Make fists with your hands and place your knuckles on your lower back. Exhale a little, then inhale as you lift your chest diagonally toward the ceiling.

8 Breathe, then return your chest and focus to look forward again by lifting through your ears. Repeat the exercise 3 more times, inhaling as you focus up toward the ceiling, and exhaling as you lengthen your spine and lift through your ears to return to look forward. As you lift your chest, feel as if a hook is pulling your breastbone up to the ceiling.

lift the chest to the ceiling

feel it here

lift through the ears to return

lift the abs toward the head

>> **lengthening** side stretch 3

9 Stand with your feet hip-width apart. Pull your navel into your spine, drop your tailbone, and bend your knees slightly. Raise your right arm and pull your right middle finger to the ceiling.

10 Look down to the left and lean and pull the left middle finger toward the floor as you reach up with the right middle finger. Elongate the whole right side of the body. Lift the pelvis (see p. 17). Take 2 breaths and then return to center. Repeat on the other side. Return to center again.

tighten
the waist

feel it here

keep the
waist tight

>> **energizing the back**

>> **articulating** compressions

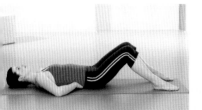

11 Lie on your back with your knees bent and the soles of your feet on the floor. Your feet should be about shoulder-width apart. Place your hands on your pubic area and abdomen to feel the movement. Compress your back sequentially into the floor: first your pubic area, then your lower back, then your mid-back. Pull your navel to your spine as you go.

hollow the
pubic area

12 Imagine you are pressing pearls into sand with your back (see p. 16) as you perform the exercise. End with a chin tuck. Hold for 4 counts, then repeat. Stretch your legs out onto the floor, and take your arms behind your head. Repeat the compressions 4 times. Relax.

tuck the chin

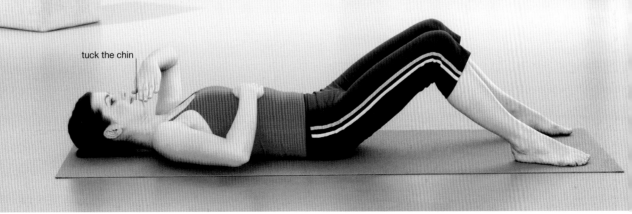

>> **coordinating** puppy dog abs

13 Lie on your back with your knees bent and arms by your sides. Hold your abdominals firm and lift your legs up so your shins are parallel to the floor. Bend your elbows, take your upper arms off the floor, and face your palms upward. This puppy dog position (see p. 17) makes your core muscles work.

take the upper arms off the floor

work the core muscles

14 Exhale, tilt your chin, lift your head, look to your groin, and lengthen your arms out past your hips. At the same time, reach your feet upward into a "V" shape, just past shoulder-width apart. Inhale and exhale, then lower back down to the puppy dog position. Repeat the exercise 3 more times.

look to the groin

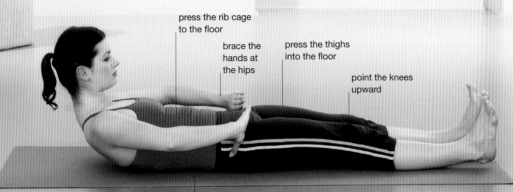

15 Lie on your back in first position parallel, with your second toe in line with your kneecaps and with the midpoint on your groin line (see p. 14). Flex your feet. Brace with your hands at your hip joint. Lift your head to check that you are in line. Keep your head up to start the exercise.

press the rib cage to the floor

brace the hands at the hips

press the thighs into the floor

point the knees upward

keep the lower back slightly off the floor

16 Exhale as you lower your head while dragging your legs to meet at the midline of your body. Firmly press your hips, knees, and ankles together, counting to 8. Repeat the lifting of your head with the opening of your legs, and the lowering of your head with pressing your legs together 3 more times. Finally, lift your head and open your legs. Relax down.

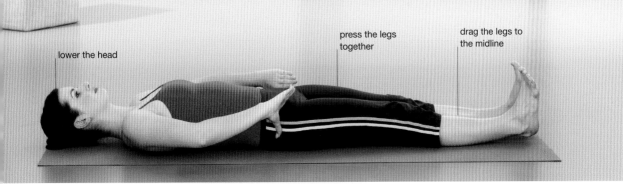

press the legs together

drag the legs to the midline

lower the head

>> **powering** hip lift

17 Lie on your right side with your right arm stretched out along the floor. Use your left hand for balance and lean up on your right forearm. Keep your legs together. Flex your feet hard and pull your toes up into your shins. Pull your navel to your spine. If balance is difficult, open your legs into a "V" shape.

press the hips forward

lean on the forearm

18 Inhale, then exhale and press downward on the legs as you look down and lift the pelvis off the floor. Hold for a moment, then lower, but not completely. Repeat 3 more times, then repeat lying on the left side.

feel it here

19 Lie on your front. Reach your hands above your head about shoulder-width apart on the floor, with your palms facing down and your arms slightly bent. Rest your forehead gently on the floor. Take your legs about 3 inches (7.5 cm) apart. Exhale, and levitate your head, hands, and feet about 2 inches (5 cm) off the floor.

pull the tailbone toward the heels

lift the abs

look downward

20 Keeping your torso as still as possible, start a small flutter-kick type of swimming motion with the feet. At the same time, "splash" alternately with your hands. Concentrate on not waddling from side to side. If your back tightens up, go down, breathe, rest, and then begin again. Work up to counting for 30 counts. Think: "1-Alligator, 2-Alligator," to set the rhythm. Relax down.

splash the hands

flutter-kick the feet

>> **stabilizing** inverted stretch

keep the right hip low

21 Go onto all fours, then tuck the toes under and lift the knees off the floor to come up into an upside-down triangle. Touching the toes of the right foot to the floor, exhale, transfer almost all your weight into the right hand, and raise the right leg up behind you.

keep the leg parallel to the floor

22 Slowly open the right leg to the right side while keeping weight in the right hand. Press into the right hand as you return the foot behind you. Give the foot a little lift, lengthen, then lower. Repeat with the left leg.

23 Stand with the legs about 3 inches (7.5 cm) apart. Place the left foot ahead of the right with about a foot's-width between the legs. The toes point forward. Cross the arms, hold the elbows, and pull the navel firmly into the spine. Reach the elbows downward.

24 Continue to reach the elbows down toward the floor. Stay in this rounded position, firmly holding the abdominals as you take 3 breaths. Carefully roll up, feeling as if the abdominals are walking up the front of the body. Repeat on the other side. Come back up and relax.

look down the length of the body

lift the pelvic muscles

engage the hollow above the pubis

energizing the back >>

15 minute **summary**

>> **energizing the back** FAQs

The Energizing the Back program contains some of the most difficult exercises in *Better Back Workout*. Beginners often cannot engage their muscles enough to know the exercises are difficult. Here are some common questions that will help you get the most from the exercises, and will explain how to modify or work up to accomplishing the hardest ones.

How do **circling motions** energize my body?

The Arm Circles require energy to stabilize the trunk. Notice the difference between circling with the rib cage loose, and again after tightening the hips, waist, and ribs. The more you lift up toward the ceiling, the more effective you'll make the exercise. The Hip Circles are similar. Moving the hips helps you find tight areas, points in the circle that are less smooth. Make a note of these and work to improve them. Wrist and Ankle Circles energize the muscles you need to balance and generate energy in little-used areas like the forearms and shins.

I don't understand the term "**compressions**." What is it I am compressing exactly?

The front of the body is soft and pliable in relation to the back, which is braced by the rib cage, the spine, and the back of the pelvis. Most people do abdominal exercise only to the point of shortening the rib cage toward the knees, but the abdominals have deep layers and there are other muscles that help to make the front of the torso concave. "Compressions" find these deeper connections that help you to go beyond traditional sit-ups.

What if my neck gets tight in the **puppy dog abs**? I find that extremely painful.

Most of the time this happens because the upper abdominals aren't engaged enough to lift the upper trunk and head. The Compressions exercise will help prepare you but if the neck still tightens, it could be due to fatigue. Then it's best to let the head come down and relax the neck. Try again after you've done the Energizing program for a couple more weeks. Your endurance will improve.

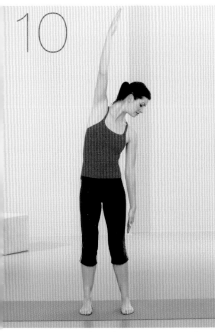

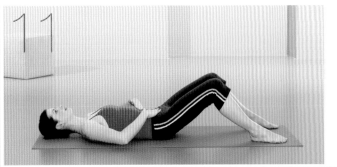

▲ **Articulating** Compressions, page 75

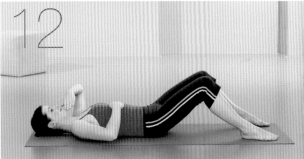

▲ **Lengthening** Side Stretch 3, page 74

▲ **Articulating** Compressions, page 75

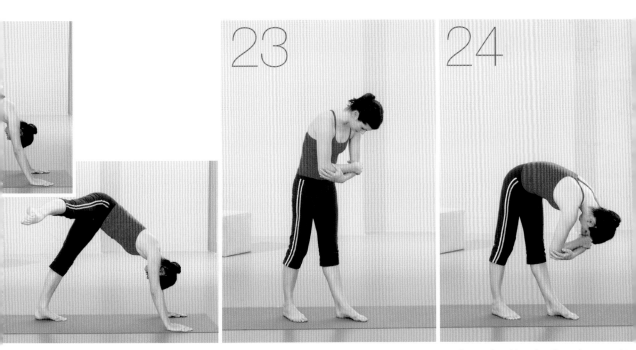

d Stretch, page 80

▲ **Centering** Hanging Stretch, page 81

▲ **Centering** Hanging Stretch, page 81

15 minute **summary**

>> ## My back tightens up in the **first position abs**. Can you suggest how can I prevent this?

The focus of this exercise is on keeping a neutral lower-back curve, which slightly elevates the lower back off the floor and makes the backs of the thighs heavy and, ideally, makes them touch the floor. If you arch and elevate the lower back too far off the floor, then bring the legs together to squeeze them, it may over-tighten the lower back. Avoid this by making sure the back of the rib cage is down against the floor. Another key point is, as you squeeze the legs together, to make sure you're tightening the inner legs near the buttocks region and not just from the front of the thighs. Squeezing from the buttocks also takes the strain off the lower back.

>> ## Can you tell me how I can prevent my calves from cramping up in the **swimming** exercise?

The body is so smart; it often accomplishes a task by using body parts other than the ones intended! This phenomenon occurs when we are doing a movement that's unfamiliar, or that may need more strength to accomplish. Prevention starts by making sure you take into account the preparatory cues before the exercise begins. Next, make the movements small instead of performing a full-fledged swimming kick. Move from the hips and keep the knees straight. One helpful image is to think of the feet as "baby feet," and keep them relaxed and not at all taut.

>> ## The **hip lift** just seems impossible. Help!

Doing exercises from the side doesn't feel natural to most people, so modify it until it feels easy. The easiest modification is to bend both knees toward the waist, lean on the forearm, and then lift the hips. The next step up is to straighten the legs, but open them. Usually I put the bottom leg forward and the top one back, being careful to keep the top hip facing up, not back. The next step is to keep both legs straight, lean onto the front hand, and then lift the hips. When you're feeling particularly macho, place the top hand on the hip, or better yet, behind the head, then lift away!

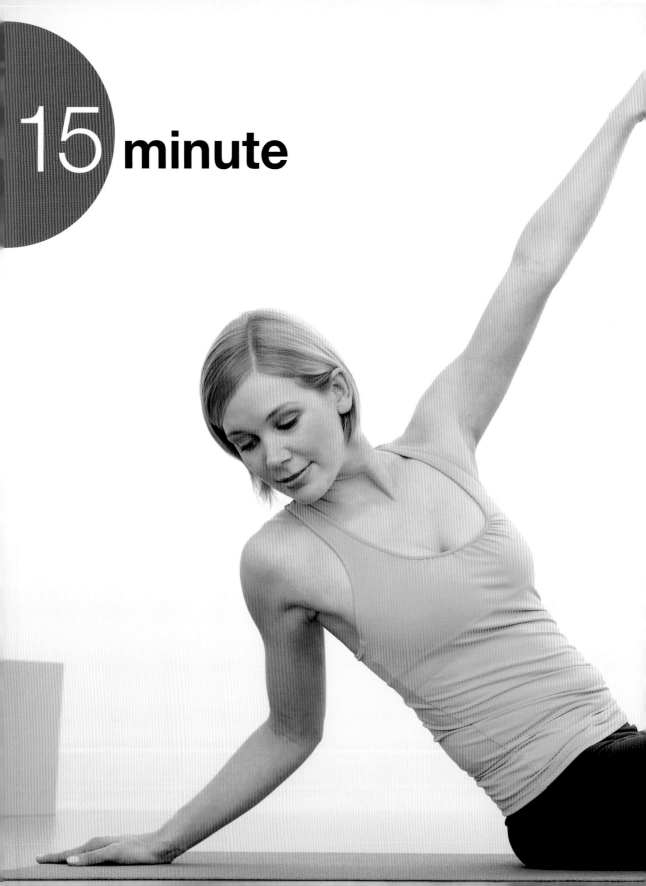

15 minute

Think supple and lithe,
smooth and flowing.
Fluidity means grace
and ease.

soothing
the back >>

>> **soothing** the back

It's a fallacy to think that the only time the back is being helped is when it's working the most strenuously. Athletes know that the best way to train is to stress the body, then relieve it, stress it, then relieve it. This final program aims to soothe and relieve, so giving the back a truly comprehensive workout.

This Soothing the Back program rounds off the four programs in my *Better Back Workout* and provides the balance that the back requires. It's possible—and desirable—to soothe your back through movement on a regular basis. While the best recipe for a healthy body is to combine both active and passive elements of care, "soothing" doesn't imply the bodily passivity of meditating, resting, and sleeping. These soothing motions are gentle but active. They help the vertebrae to achieve a better range of motion, and optimally to operate in a flowing manner. It is said that we are only as young as our spines. A youthful, healthy spine moves without stiffness from bone to bone. The exercises in this final program are designed particularly to promote fluidity. They help us to achieve the goal of moving effortlessly and with grace and ease throughout our daily tasks.

The exercises

Set the tone for the exercises in this program by starting with the Cat and Camel, a classic back exercise. Unleash the power of the program by focusing on elongating. Avoid the pitfall of simply hinging the spine at its primary hinge point—the waist. Instead, imagine the head is pulling forward in opposition to the backward pull of the tail. Round up into the breastbone and reach all the points of the bones of the spine up and away from the floor. Once you've become sensitive to all the different parts of the spine, keep their image in your mind as you go into the next exercises.

> ## >>**tips for** soothing the back
>
> - **Think of your spine as a long snake** and see it in your mind as very supple and lithe.
>
> - **Note any choppy** or incomplete movements as you go through these exercises. Try to keep all your movements super-smooth.
>
> - **As you repeat the exercises,** strive to make the motions even smoother, like silk sliding over glass.
>
> - **Note particularly** how comfortable you are as you move from one direction to the other in Rounded Alligator and Baby Rolls.

The elongated spine image will help you with the more difficult Combined Curl-up. If the neck gets tight, lower it and elongate the neck as if someone were pulling it gently away from the torso. The Seated "U" challenges the elongated spine in sitting and leaning; the Heel Taps challenge it while lying on the stomach. To modify the Forearm Plank, simply lower the knees onto the ground instead of straightening them all the way.

Soothe the back with this gentle program. Use it as a starting point if you are new to exercise, to give variety to your workouts, and at times when you need restoration.

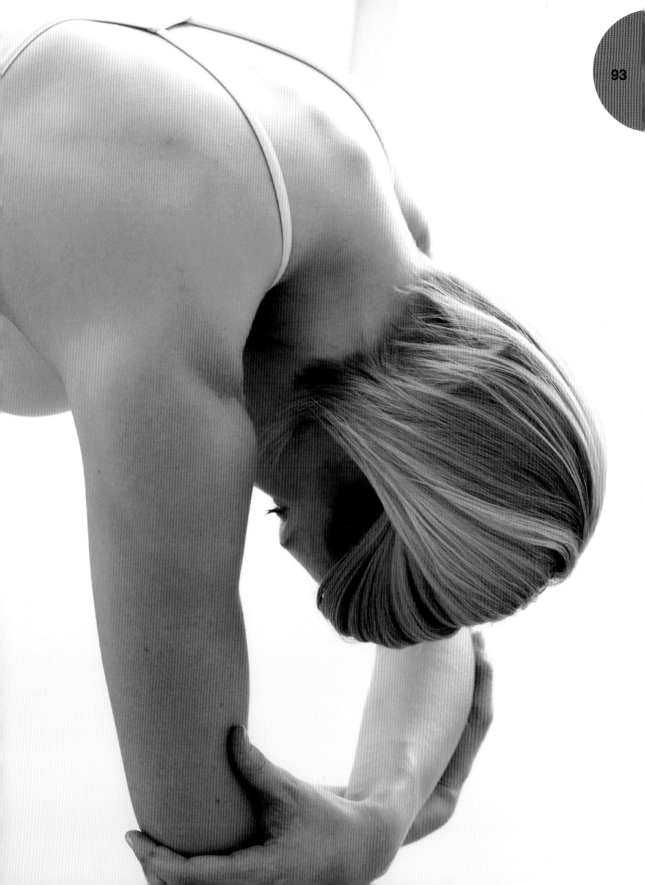

>> **elongating** cat and camel

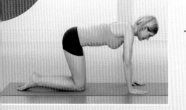

1 Start on all fours with your back flat in the tabletop position (see p. 16). Lengthen out from your tailbone as though you have a long tail. Then reach out through your head and tilt your chin and tailbone down at the same time. Round your back to look at your navel, like a scared cat.

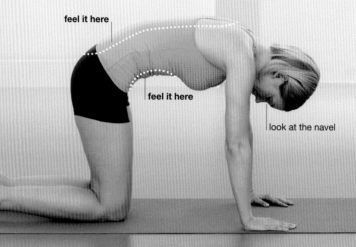

feel it here

feel it here

look at the navel

2 Exhale and lengthen back to the tabletop, then look forward and arch your back like a camel by reaching up and out through your head. Feel as if your tailbone could reach the top of your head. Repeat the exercise 1 more time. Return to the tabletop position and relax.

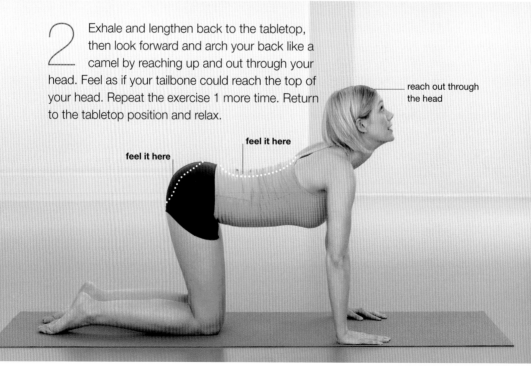

reach out through the head

feel it here

feel it here

>> **coordinating** rounded alligator

3 Remain on all fours and look toward your right hip.
Swing your right hip toward your right shoulder.
Now round your back and look at your navel as in
the scared cat position (see opposite).

look at the navel

4 Repeat the exercise to look at the left hip,
while swinging the left hip toward the left
shoulder. Round the back again and look
at the navel. Repeat 2 more times.

swing the left hip to
the left shoulder

>> **articulating** baby rolls

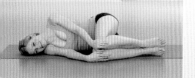

5 Start by lying on your right side with your legs bent up. Hold your hands on top of your knees. Put a towel around your neck if you need extra support. Roll onto your back, feeling as much of your back as possible resting against the floor.

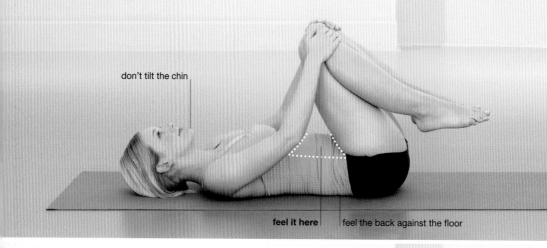

don't tilt the chin

feel it here | feel the back against the floor

6 Then roll over onto your left side, letting your focus and head linger to the right. Think: "leg, leg," then head rolls last. Repeat the exercise, starting on your left side, then rolling onto your back, and lingering the focus to the left. Continue gently rolling from side to side 3 more times.

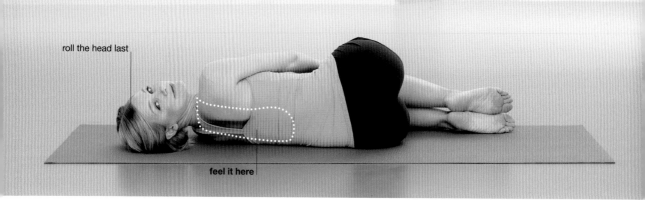

roll the head last

feel it here

>> **softening** sacral circles

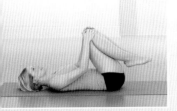

7 Roll to your back with your knees bent. Compress your abdomen thoroughly to touch all parts of your back to the floor. Hold onto your knees. Then gently circle your knees together. Feel as though you are circling the rim of a saucer with your pelvis. Circle in both directions 2 times.

compress the abdomen | circle the pelvis

8 Place the soles of your feet on the floor. Keep your knees bent. Place your hands on your hip bones for feedback. Circle your pelvis again as before. Move in one direction for 4 circles, then reverse. Circle your pelvis 2 more times in each direction.

place hands
on hip bones

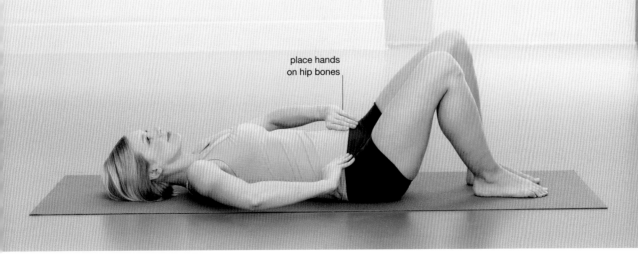

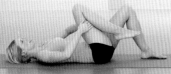

pull the toes
toward the shin

feel it here

9 Stay on your back. Bend both knees. Take your feet about 4 inches (10 cm) apart. Lift up your right leg and use both hands to hold loosely behind your lifted thigh. Then gently straighten your knee. It does not have to straighten completely. At the top of the stretch, pull your toes toward your shin.

10 Still holding onto the thigh, bend the knee, letting the foot come down so the shin makes a parallel line with the floor. Perform this pumping action 10 times. Repeat the exercise holding the left leg. Relax.

bring the shin
parallel with the floor

>> **centering** inverse frog

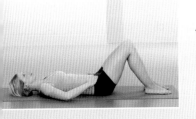

11 Stay on your back with bent knees. Compress your whole back against the floor and place your hands on your hips for feedback. Keep your back pressed firmly against the floor as you gently open both knees sideways toward the floor, like a frog. Let the soles of your feet come together.

place hands
on hip bones

soles of the feet
come together

feel the back against the floor

12 Exhale and deepen the abdominal compression as you bring the knees together again. Repeat the froglike opening and closing 3 more times. Relax.

bring the knees
together

compress the
abdomen

press the lower back against the floor

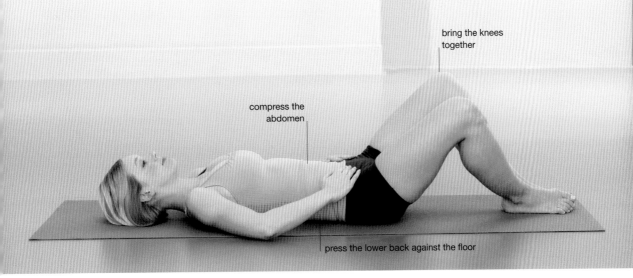

>> **articulating** ballooning

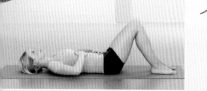

13 Stay on your back with knees bent. Let your whole back fall into the floor. Place your left hand on your abdomen, and your right hand on your rib cage with your thumb between your breasts. Breathe in through your nose. Expand your chest and tighten your abdominals.

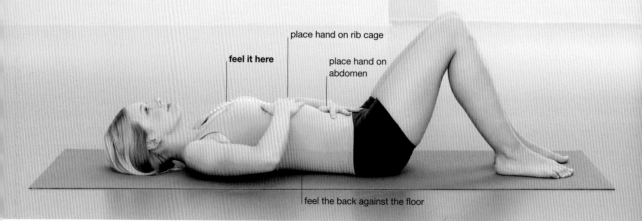

place hand on rib cage

feel it here

place hand on abdomen

feel the back against the floor

14 Now reverse the action. Breathe out through your mouth, squeeze your chest, and expand your abdominals. Inhale, expand your chest; exhale, and squeeze your chest, for 3 more repetitions. Think of mercury in a thermometer flowing up and down the front of your spine as you perform this exercise.

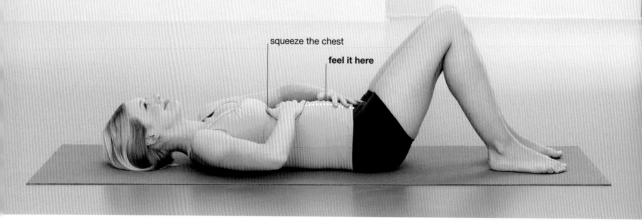

squeeze the chest

feel it here

15 Stay on the back with knees bent and heels lifted, a little apart. Clasp the hands behind the head. Simultaneously tilt the chin, curl the upper body off the floor to look at the groin, and tuck and roll the tailbone off the floor. Imagine a dog's tail between the legs, lifting the tailbone and spine (see p17).

imagine keeping
the ribs below
the tailbone

16 Take a breath, then lower your head, shoulders and tailbone back down to the ground at the same time. Keep your heels up off the floor. Imagine you are pressing pearls into sand with your spine (see p16). Repeat the Combined Curl-up 2 more times.

keep the elbows out

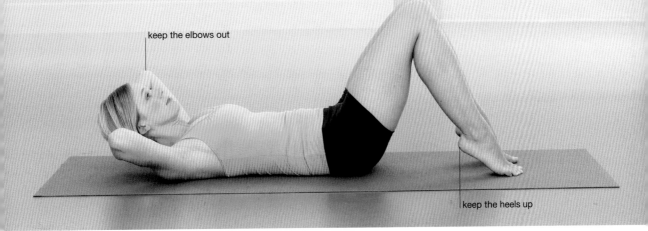

keep the heels up

>> **balancing** seated "U"

17 Sit up tall on your sitbones with both legs extended straight out in front of you. Feel an imaginary hand lifting the skin of your lower back up and toward your head. Then pull your toes up toward your shins, exhale, and levitate your hands to make a "U" shape.

drop the shoulders down

reach out with the top hand

18 Keeping your back straight, reach back with your right arm. Bend your elbow, lean back, and simultaneously look to your right. Then quickly lift back up with your arms to the "U" shape. Repeat to the other side. Alternate the leaning and lifting from side to side for 3 more sets.

>> soothing the back

>> **accentuating** heel taps

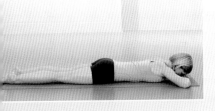

19 Lie on your front with outstretched legs. Place your hands underneath your forehead, and rest your head on top. Rotate your legs to a "V" shape, heels together and toes apart. Exhale as you levitate your head, hands, and feet about 2 inches (5 cm) off the floor. Feel the smile lines (see p. 16). Look downward.

take the tailbone
toward the heels

lift the abs

20 Tap the heels together a total of 32 times, in 4 sets of 8. Frequently improve the work of the exercise by holding the abdominals inward and tight, anchoring the hips with a strong tailbone tuck, and pulling the gaze toward the floor. End by holding and tightening the hips, then lower down and relax.

regularly check
the abs are tight

>> **powering** forearm plank

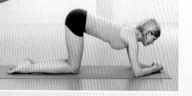

21 Go onto the forearms and knees. Clasp the hands in front of you. Feel imaginary hands sandwiching the waist (see p. 17). One lifts the abdominal contents and the other gently presses down on the lower back. Inhale and exhale to reach the right foot and then the left behind you to create a forearm plank.

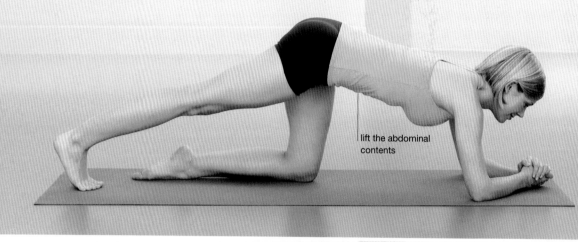

lift the abdominal contents

22 Pull up the abdominals and press the pubic bone down toward the floor. Curl the tailbone under to firmly lock in the hips. Take 2 breaths. Bend the knees back to kneeling, then repeat the exercise. Relax.

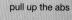

pull up the abs

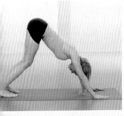

23 From all fours, exhale and lift the hips, holding the navel to the spine (see p. 17). Walk the hands toward the feet. Keep the knees a little bent. Take 2 breaths, then start rolling up. As you pass the thighs, cross the wrists and take off an imaginary shirt.

24 Continue rolling up, feeling as if the vertebrae are stacking up vertically through the lower back, waistline, rib cage, and shoulders, until the head reaches up on top of the pelvis (see p. 17). Circle the arms to lower. Relax.

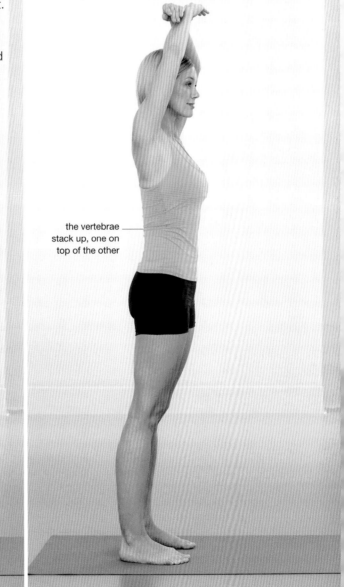

the vertebrae stack up, one on top of the other

feel how the head becomes heavy

feel how the tailbone becomes heavy

soothing the back >>

15 minute **summary**

>> **soothing the back** FAQs

Soothing your back is possible through exercise. The body is designed to move in a myriad of ways and varying the type of exercise you perform provides balance. This Soothing the Back program offers a kinder and gentler form of movement. Its soothing exercises accentuate the quality of motion, making your movements smooth and effortless.

>> ## I don't understand how the **baby rolls** will help my back. Can you explain please?

The Baby Rolls promote what we call "mature" motion of the spine. A fully developed body is capable of moving in all directions. When you roll from side to side, with the head rolling last, you effectively rotate the entire spine. So Baby Rolls help you to achieve a full rotational range of movement in all the segments of the spine. I do this exercise daily to keep my spine healthy.

>> ## What do **sacral circles** do?

They do several things. They help to stretch all parts of the waist, especially in the back, in the tough tissues between the ribs and the pelvis. These tissues often become unbalanced by one part being too short and the other too long. Sacral Circles are also a great abdominal toner. The abdominals contain several layers of muscles, and Sacral Circles hit them all.

>> ## How do the **knee pumps** build a better back?

Knee Pumps are really an exercise to make the sciatic nerve—the large nerve that runs down the back of the thigh from the pelvis—stretch more easily and if the area around the pelvis is comfortable, that will help the back, too. Nerves stretch at a different rate than the muscles; sometimes leg tightness is really a sciatic nerve tightness and not muscle tightness. Knee Pumps also relieve back tension and "oil" the knee joints so they're happier.

What does **ballooning** do?

Ballooning is the sneakiest of the torso exercises because it is a wonderful toner for both the abdomen and the diaphragm. The diaphragm divides the torso into two cavities—the thoracic cavity in the rib cage and the abdominal cavity in the abdomen. Ballooning effectively stretches these two areas from the inside out. It is as if you are squeezing one side of a balloon and seeing the other side bulge. Since you use muscles to activate the motion, you also get this wonderful abdominal and diaphragmatic toning effect.

How does the **seated "U"** help the back?

It works on the back because it makes you lean away from your center of gravity. One aspect of balance and core training is to destabilize your base of support, which here is your hips. As you lean back, your muscles "grab" because the body intuitively knows that it's falling off balance. Then those muscles activate more to bring you back to a balanced position. The back has more muscles than any other part of the body, so getting them all activated and toned presents a challenge. The Seated "U" hits many of these muscles.

 ## The **heel taps** feel awkward and I find that my legs don't come together at the same time. Can you tell me what that's about?

Lying prone on the stomach is the most unnatural, and so the most awkward, position for people since they usually sit and stand all day. Babies go through a period of lying on their stomachs in order to develop strong enough back muscles to stand, and we are the same. Comprehensive back-strengthening programs must always include prone-lying exercises. The tapping of the heels creates an added challenge because the limbs are moving. Tapping together at the same time forces us to negotiate and smooth out any discrepancies in side-to-side (right-to-left) back and inner-thigh movement.

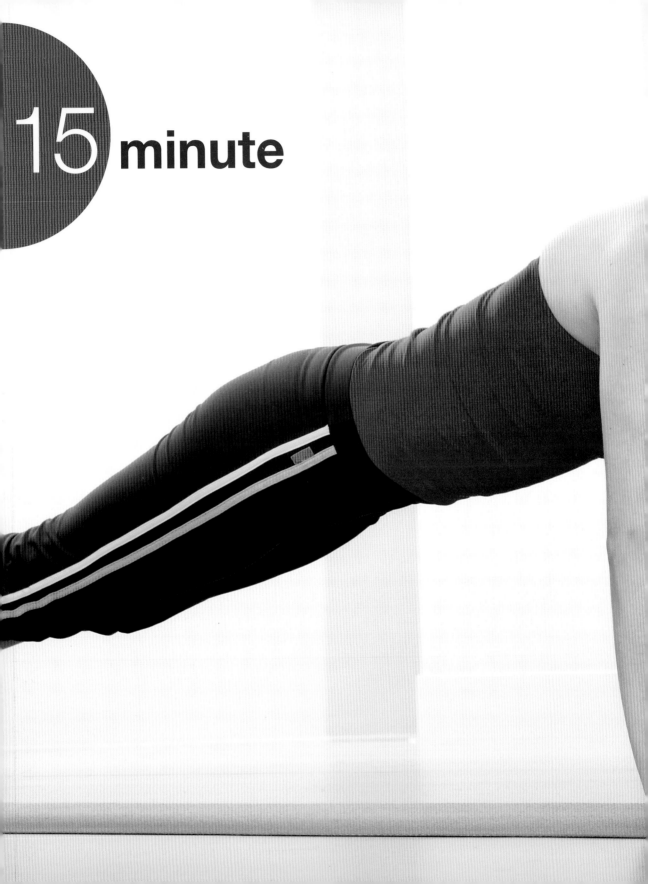

15 minute

Progress your exercise
work. Stay motivated.
Find a class. Lead a
healthy lifestyle.

moving on
from here >>

>> **how to** make progress

Progression often seems tricky but you just have to get started and suspend judgment about how you are doing. Try to follow the instructions as faithfully as you can, bearing in mind the imagery, pacing, and cue guidance. Once you are familar with the exercises, you can begin to ramp-up your program.

Familiarize yourself with all four programs before beginning any exercise. The programs are all designed so they begin slowly and gently and work up to become more difficult. If you are a complete beginner, try starting with Soothing the Back.

Whatever your level of fitness, you should be able to do most of the 12 exercises in each of the programs, especially those of the Soothing the Back program. If you cannot do all the exercises, be proud for the ones you have completed. It is never a failing to skip an exercise that makes you uncomfortable, or that your body tells you you should not be attempting.

To make the exercise easier if you need, bend your knees or do only part. Be smart and allow yourself some variation until you feel you can do the exercises as demonstrated. Aim to do the workout three times per week and expect to be a bit sore. Soreness is natural on the first day after beginning new exercises, and peaks on the second day. Soon your body will be trained to expect a daily dose of physical exertion. Then progress by taking the advice below for the occasional exerciser.

Occasional exercisers

If you are an occasional exerciser, start with the Developing the Back program three times a week for two weeks. Then progress to the Revitalizing the Back, Energizing the Back, and Soothing the Back programs in that order for two weeks each. That way you'll teach your body to accept a variety of movements and stresses from many directions,

> >> **tips for** making progress
>
> - **Novices** and people recovering from illness should start with Soothing the Back three times a week.
>
> - **Occasional exercisers** should start with Developing the Back three times a week for two weeks, then progress the other programs in a six-week cycle.
>
> - **Regular exercisers** should randomize the programs, starting with Developing the Back. Daily back workouts are best.
>
> - **To progress to a full one-hour workout,** first pair the Soothing program with the Developing program, then add the others, one at a time, when you are able to do so.

plus you'll complete a solid eight-week conditioning program that is sure to get you noticed for your erect posture and stance. Have faith and persist if you only have time to be an occasional exerciser. The benefits of a strong back and better posture will creep up on you!

Regular exercisers

If you exercise regularly, then randomize the order of the programs from the very outset. I recommend starting with Developing the Back. Performing a program once a day will give wonderful results. Remember that all these exercises are safe to perform on consecutive days.

Doubling up the programs is a great way to fast-track your progress. Try pairing Developing the Back with Soothing the Back for two weeks, three times per week, and then progress to pairing Revitalizing and Energizing with the Soothing program in that order for another four weeks.

One-hour workout

You can also gradually work up to doing all four sequences at once to give a one-hour workout. Use the Regular exercisers strategy above, then slowly double and triple the workouts until you achieve all four at once. When you reach this point, remember to factor in some recovery time, taking two consecutive days off every few weeks.

Problem backs

If you are recovering from a back condition or major illness, check with your medical practitioner before using the *Better Back Workout*. The Soothing the Back program will be best to begin with. Start with several repetitions of the Cat and Camel, Rounded Alligator, and Sacral Circles, and slowly progress to the full program. Even if you were an advanced exerciser before your illness, start slowly, picking the exercises that come easiest. If you truly can't complete a number of them, try imagining in as detailed a fashion as you can that you are exercising. Research reveals that just doing this can activate the connections between brain and body.

If you have a problem back, doing several repetitions of the gentle Cat and Camel is a safe and gentle way to start getting used to exercising your back.

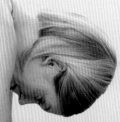

>> **staying** motivated

Staying the course to achieve your goals is a well-researched subject. You can train yourself into a new behavior, using conscious effort, in about 21 to 28 days. After that, maintaining your selected program becomes more automatic, and eventually can become a real lifestyle change.

To begin with, you need to commit yourself to three weeks to push through the initial unfamiliarity of the programs. This will lay the ground for further benefit. *Better Back Workout* will give maximum advantage if you select one program to do at least three days per week. However, all four of the *Better Back Workout* programs can certainly be done daily, even more than once, if you wish. I perform many of the exercises in the program about five days per week to keep my back strong.

After the first three weeks

After your initial three weeks, you may encounter "bumps in the road." This is where novelty and variation come in. A comprehensive fitness program involves cardiovascular work such as walking, bicycling, and swimming in order to give the heart and lungs a workout. Alternating your *Better Back Workout* programs with this type of activity will keep you fresh for more.

Working toward a progress benchmark is another great way to stay on track. A benchmark can be as simple as managing to perform one program four times a week for the first three weeks, or just realizing that sitting at your computer has suddenly become easier. My clients frequently keep a small exercise journal to chart their frequency of exercise, and what their achievements are.

Keep in mind that there is no way you can lose; faithfully giving positive attention to yourself can give only positive results. At first the movements may seem foreign and uncomfortable. You may not

> ## >>**tips for** staying motivated
>
> - **Commit yourself to three weeks** to push through the unfamiliarity barrier.
>
> - **Introduce variety,** alternating the programs with other exercise that you can easily fit into your routine—walking or cycling are good examples.
>
> - **Work toward a progress benchmark,** such as aiming to perform one sequence four nights a week for the first three weeks.
>
> - **Keep an exercise journal** to chart the frequency of your exercise and the goals you want to achieve each week.

even be able to do one or two of the exercises. Don't give up. Visualize your healthy body and use the models as your guide to help you perform the sequences to the best of your ability.

Some days you'll feel better than others. If you persist, you will often find that just going through a program will make you feel better on a down day. As I tell my clients, once you make exercise part of your routine, you'll begin to crave it!

Get yourself into a routine where you try to train at the same time each day, if possible. You'll quickly gain a sense of satisfaction each time you unroll that exercise mat.

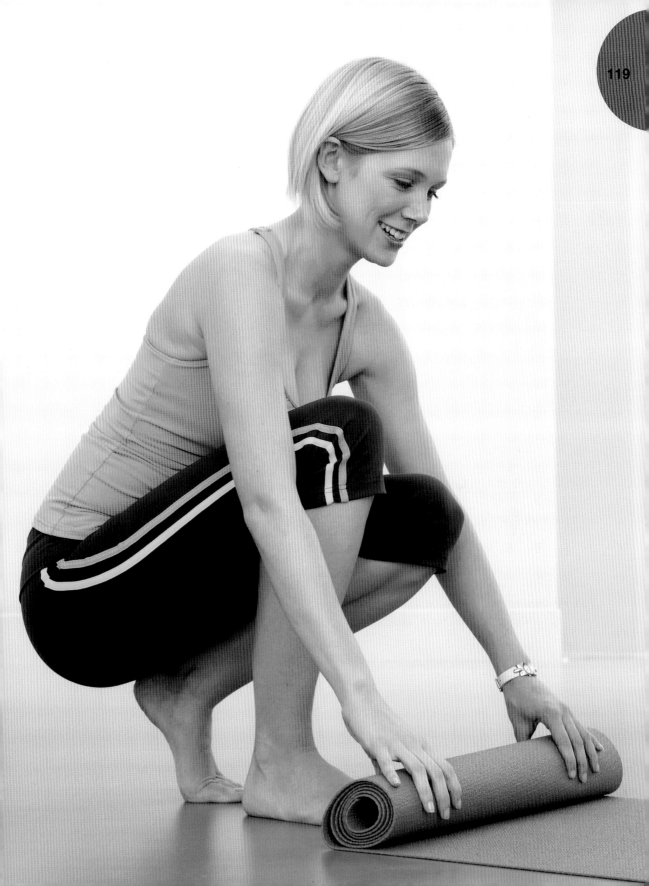

>> **finding** a teacher

Congratulations on working your way through my *Better Back Workout*! Now you may well want to know about how to find full-hour group classes and private instructors who can help you with your progress and also individualize challenges and goals for you that are tailored to your needs.

Finding a teacher mostly takes keeping your eyes open. The familiarity with exercising that you have gained by using my *Better Back Workout* will help you compare the type of material that is offered in classes and the way that content is presented to you. Be careful of simply being drawn in by the charisma of an attractive and fit instructor. First decide if you want a stretch class, a movement class such as cardio-fusion, a fun and funky class like hip-hop or street dance, or an inner-focused mind–body class, such as yoga offers.

Content is essential, yet many people select their exercise classes strictly from class titles and are not savvy when it comes to analyzing the content. A far better way to see what you're getting into is to observe the class. Watch and see if the instructor looks at the participants or is simply in love with the image in the mirror. Watch also to see that he or she is neither overzealous, in which case they risk causing injury, nor ineffective, which will be a waste of your money and time.

Check the instructor's qualifications

Ask for the teacher's credentials, such as certifications or college degrees. There is no need for an uneducated teacher. Instructors now have the resources to become educated in basic body mechanics and general health. You deserve to be reassured that your instructor is properly trained and qualified. If a teacher says he or she is self-educated and doesn't need formal training, remember that is a code for "quack."

> ## >> **tips for** finding a teacher
>
> - **Select classes based on** observation, not just class titles.
>
> - **Notice if the teacher** watches the students, and note the interactions between the teacher and the students.
>
> - **Beware of the charismatic teacher,** who teaches on personality alone, without thought to safety or content. Chemistry counts, but there has to be more.
>
> - **Become a regular attendee.** The teacher will be able to observe and guide you best if they are able to watch you over time.

If you have a special back issue, do have a brief chat with the instructor before deciding to join that class. Get an idea if the instructor is hesitant about your participation. Also be aware that the instructor may be warning you that the class is not for you, and heed the advice. Usually a teacher will have ideas about other classes that may be better for your body type, fitness level, or rehabilitation needs.

Going to class with a friend—the buddy system—can help in getting you to a class, but if for some reason it is not the right class for you, you will be going backward. If you have to go to a certain class because you need a ride with a friend, but you find that though the content is right, your chemistry is not right with the instructor, don't throw out the baby with the bath water. Figure out what you need and attempt a little negotiation. Being assertive in a nonconfrontational manner can help both you and your instructor.

Once you've embarked on a class, do give it time, since only time will tell if you've found your mentor. Just like job interviews, you may have to go through 10 instructors to find that special one. However, if the instructor is anything less than respectful and encouraging toward you, go and find another class, no matter how much you feel you want to belong to that particular group. Of course, class dynamics will vary from lesson to lesson, but every class should make you walk away saying to yourself, "Every day in every way, I'm getting better and better!"

One of the best ways to fast-track your progress is to work with your class teacher privately, even if it's only for a few sessions. This will aid you in understanding your progression rate, and will help to demystify more of the language and concepts you will come across as you go on.

Matching your goals to a class and instructor may take more time and effort than you expected. Just mentioning what you are looking for in a class when you show up for the first time may not make the class what you intended. An attentive instructor will prepare classes with the regulars in mind, not the newcomers, though he or she should encourage and help new participants find their way.

Remember that everybody needs something different. Finding a class and teacher that are right for you will bring you satisfaction, fellowship, and improvement beyond your expectations.

Finding a teacher takes footwork, asking friends for references, and being patient while exploring the options. The right teacher will help you with your specific goals.

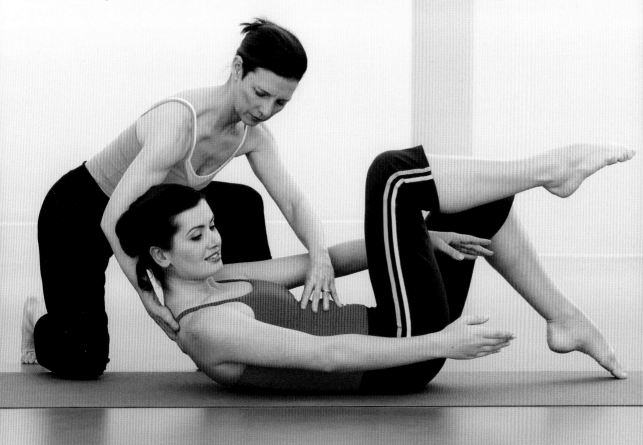

>> **healthy** living

Once you start to feel the benefits of *Better Back Workout*, you will certainly take a more holistic interest in your body. That means thinking not just about exercise, but also about nutrition, rest, and restoration. Ensuring this balance makes life worth living and allows us to remain happy along the way!

"Rest, digest, and heal" is one of my favorite mantras. Everyone needs rest, nutrition, and restoration, from the most active athletes and physical laborers to the busiest, most stressed-out mom or office worker. The winning formula invariably involves alternating periods of activity and stimulation with periods of rest and relaxation. Eating the right foods, in the appropriate amounts, and establishing a regular sleep schedule are additional invaluable tools that help to promote overall wellbeing and lifelong happiness.

We live in a wonderful time when food, for those of us in the developed world, is abundant. Science and research now provide young and old alike with specific information about what nutrients they need, how food is metabolized in the body, and what foods are beneficial, and why. Eating fresh foods, including antioxidant foods, watching the sugar content in our fruits and vegetables, and monitoring the amount of water in our daily diet are strategies that pay off when it comes to focusing on a better back. These strategies help us maintain an appropriate weight for our height, which is crucial in not challenging the back more than it needs. Having a pot belly and carrying extra poundage literally places severe, unnecessary, and dangerous loads on the spine.

>>**tips for** healthy living

- **Choose five servings** of fruits and vegetables per day.

- **Include protein-rich** foods in your diet for better health and a better back, too.

- **Limit your intake of alcohol,** high-sugar and high-fat foods.

- **Drink at least** six glasses of water per day.

- **Match your carbohydrate level** to your level of activity.

- **Alternate activity with rest,** even if the rest periods can only be brief.

Remember the 80/20 rule: If you eat well and rest well 80 percent of the time, you can eat whatever you like for the remaining 20 percent!

Nutrition essentials

Our bodies require the basic nutrients provided by carbohydrates, fats, and proteins. Hydration is also an essential requirement of all living things. Carbohydrates are vegetables, fruits, and starches. Starches are heavy carbohydrates like bread, potatoes, and pasta. The carbohydrates all provide energy and vitamins. Good fats, such as mono-unsaturated fats and omega-3 oils, are necessary for the hormones—the chemical messengers that regulate reproduction, the metabolism, and bone functions among others—and for our skin, which is our primary immune defense system.

Last but not least are the proteins—the building blocks that make up the ligamentous and muscular systems that bind the joints together. To have a better back, you particularly need sufficient protein, since the back alone is made up of over 50 joints. Providing adequate amounts of protein for the constant repair that a moving, living spine requires demands special attention. Protein-rich foods are nuts, lean meats, seafood, whole grains, and legumes such as peas and beans.

Sleep requirements

Modern life often means sleep loss. Getting six to eight hours regularly can be challenging for new parents, students, commuters, and avid television viewers. The fourth stage of sleep is most important. It is when our tissues heal from the knocks and overuse of everyday living, and it enables us to cope with our everyday stresses to boot. Backs are particularly vulnerable to stress, fatigue, and remaining upright for extended periods. Attending to proper rest, in a horizontal position, lessens the strains of gravity on the joints as well as lessening our emotional burdens.

Overtraining and overstimulation are also detrimental. Overtraining causes an inability to sleep and that's when injuries increase dramatically. Everyone loves the occasional night out, but ongoing overstimulation eventually causes burnout. The humbling truth is that our bodies— and our backs—are finite. They, like us, need regular rest and restoration.

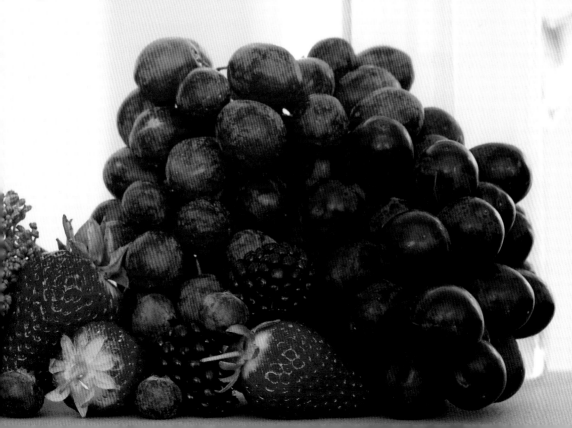

useful resources

It is always best to seek medical advice from medical professionals regarding back problems. However, it is also prudent to take a proactive approach to general health and preventative care. These resources will help you find professionals, and general information.

General fitness resources

The American College of Sports Medicine
www.acsm.org
ACSM promotes and integrates scientific research, education, and practical applications of sports medicine and exercise science to maintain and enhance physical performance, fitness, health, and quality of life.

The American Council on Exercise
www.acefitness.org
ACE is a nonprofit organization committed to enriching quality of life through safe and effective physical activity. ACE protects all segments of society against ineffective fitness products, programs, and trends through its ongoing public education, outreach, and research. ACE further protects the public by setting certification and continuing education standards for fitness professionals.

General physical therapy resources

The American Physical Therapy Association
www.APTA.org
The mission of the American Physical Therapy Association (APTA), the principal membership organization representing and promoting the profession of physical therapy, is to further the profession's role in the prevention, diagnosis, and treatment of movement dysfunctions and the enhancement of the physical health and functional abilities of members of the public.

PEDro (Physiotherapy Evidence Database)
A web-based database of randomized controlled trials and systematic reviews in physiotherapy. It can be accessed free of charge at: www.pedro.fhs.usyd.edu.au/

Professional and studio resources for Pilates

The Pilates Method is well known for offering core conditioning and back rehabilitation and has been proven to help with lower back stabilization. Yoga and the Feldenkreis Method are also useful for the back, particularly to increase range of motion, but the primary focus of the Pilates Method is strengthening and stabilization of the spine. For this reason, as a Pilates practitioner for over 20 years, I believe that the principles and concepts of the Pilates Method can be applied to all physicality involving the back. The exercises in *Better Back Workout* are largely influenced by the Pilates Method.

Pilates Method Alliance
www.pilatesmethodalliance.org
The PMA is an international organization that seeks to keep the Pilates Method pure. It is the gold-standard in the certification of the Pilates Method, and is a great resource for finding studios and teachers in your location.

Pilates Therapeutics

www.pilatestherapeutics.com
I founded Pilates Therapeutics in 2001 to combine the art of therapy, movement principles, and the Pilates Method, in an accessible way for both health-care providers and the public. The Pilates Therapeutics mission is to illuminate how the concepts of the Pilates Method can be adapted for therapeutic use. It also aims to motivate the public to embark on the hopeful path of finding solutions to musculo-skeletal problems, and to alleviate pain and unnecessary suffering through education and the management of common conditions such as scoliosis, repetitive stress injuries, and breast cancer.

Websites for specific back-related ailments

National Scoliosis Foundation
www.scoliosis.org

Arthritis Foundation
www.arthritis.org

DVDs by Suzanne Martin

The Upper Core: Exercises for Repetitive Stress Injuries of the Upper Body
(Pilates Therapeutics® 2002)
The Upper Core was developed to respond to the prevalence of repetitive stress injuries of the shoulders, arms, and hands that have accompanied our increased use of computers. This DVD provides 25 excellent restorative and corrective exercises for any upper-extremity problem, ranging from computer overuse to surgery to cancer.

The Pelvic Ring Core: Exercises for Pelvic and Leg Imbalances
(Pilates Therapeutics® 2002)
The Pelvic Ring Core focuses on 24 balancing exercises to help lower back and pelvic pain, knee problems, and post-pregnancy restoration. It is excellent for strengthening the smaller muscles that can help people regain their larger muscle activities, such as biking, running, and dancing.

The Scoliosis Management Series

Part 1: A Wall–Spring Home Exercise Program
(Pilates Therapeutics® 2006)
Part 1 is designed to help people who have scoliosis or abnormal curvature of the spine. Instructions for using Wall Springs as a home-exercise program and for screening for significant scoliosis with a Scoliometer® are included, together with core-control exercises and a 30-minute exercise "flow."

Part 2: Breathing Exercises
(Pilates Therapeutics® 2007)
Part 2 continues the concepts for managing scoliosis of *Part 1* (see above), but focuses on breathing for long-term management. It includes simple instructions on how to measure your lung volume and improve your breathing capacity, together with a 20-minute guided exercise "flow" to improve chest and rib cage range of motion.

A Step-Wise Approach to Post-Natal Restoration
(Pilates Therapeutics® 2007)
This is designed to be of use to any woman who has given birth in the last 18 months or who will shortly give birth. Sections include exercises for foot strengthening, instructions for therapeutic contrast baths (alternation of hot then cold baths), corrective exercises for post-natal distended abdomen, and a 25-minute guided exercise "flow" for daily practice.

A Breast Cancer Survivor's Guide to Physical Restoration
(Pilates Therapeutics® 2007)
This is for women who have had or will have surgery related to breast-cancer treatment. Sections include core control, corrective exercises after transverse abdominal or latissimus dorsi flap procedures, lymphedema education and control, scar softening and reduction, skin care, a survivors' guided 30-minute exercise "flow" for weekly practice, and a comprehensive guide to the resumption of fitness activites.

to contact Suzanne Martin
www.totalbodydevelopment.com

index

acknowledgments

Author's acknowledgments

Thank you to so many who made this project possible. What luck to have the wonderful design of Miranda Harvey, the attentiveness of Hilary Mandleberg, the exquisite photography of Ruth Jenkinson, and thanks especially to Penny Warren and Mary-Clare Jerram for making *Better Back Workout* happen. I am deeply grateful to models Rhona and Sam for their concentration and physical perseverance, and the behind-the-scenes DK staff who pulled together every detail also deserve a tip of the hat. Thanks also for question ideas from the staff of Smuin Ballet, Joellen Arntz, Vincent Avery, Kaleena Opdyke, and dancer Aaron Thayer. A special thanks to Leilani Lau for playful pelvic images and much-appreciated technical support. And last, a big kiss of appreciation to my patient, loving husband, Tom Martin.

Publisher's acknowledgments

Dorling Kindersley would like to thank photographer Ruth Jenkinson and her assistants, James McNaught and Vic Churchill; sweatyBetty for the loan of the exercise clothing; Viv Riley at Touch Studios; the models Rhona Crewe and Sam Johannesson; Roisin Donaghy and Victoria Barnes for the hair and makeup; YogaMatters for supplying the mat.

about Suzanne Martin

Suzanne is a doctor of physical therapy and a gold-certified Pilates expert. A former dancer, she is a Master trainer certified by the American Council on Exercise. She is published by *Dance Magazine*, Dorling Kindersley, and the *Journal of Dance Medicine and Science*, among others. She is also well known as an educational presenter within the world of Pilates, dance, and physical therapy. Suzanne is the lead physical therapist for the Smuin Ballet in San Francisco and maintains a private practice, Total Body Development, in Alameda, California.

For more information, check her website www.totalbodydevelopment.com.